NEUROLOGICAL
EXAMINATION
MADE EASY

For Churchill Livingstone

Publisher: Michael Parkinson
Project Editor: Dilys Jones
Copy Editor: Susan Hunter
Production Controller: Lesley Small
Sales Promotion Executive: Duncan Jones

NEUROLOGICAL EXAMINATION
MADE EASY

Geraint Fuller MA MD MRCP
Senior Registrar,
Charing Cross Hospital,
London,
UK

Illustrations by
Matthew Gale MA PhD

CHURCHILL LIVINGSTONE
EDINBURGH LONDON MADRID MELBOURNE NEW YORK TOKYO 1993

CHURCHILL LIVINGSTONE
Medical Division of Longman Group UK Limited

Distributed in the United States of America by Churchill
Livingstone Inc., 650 Avenue of the Americas, New York, N.Y. 10011,
and by associated companies, branches and representatives
throughout the world.

First published 1993
  Reprinted 1994 (twice)

ISBN 0-443-04294-2

British Library of Cataloguing in Publication Data
A catalogue record for this book is available from the British Library.

Library of Congress Cataloging in Publication Data
Fuller, Geraint.
    Neurological examination made easy/Geraint Fuller;
illustrations by Matthew Gate.
        p.   cm.
    Includes bibliographical references and index.
    ISBN 0–443–04294–2
    1. Neurological examination. I. Title.
    [DNLM: 1. Neurologic Examination. WL 141 F965n]
RC348.F85 1993
616.8′0475—dc20
DNLM/DLC
for Library of Congress   92-48187

The
publisher's
policy is to use
**paper manufactured
from sustainable forests**

Produced by Longman Singapore Publishers (Pte) Ltd
Printed in Singapore

CONTENTS

ACKNOWLEDGEMENTS

I would like to thank all my teachers, particularly Dr Roberto Guiloff who introduced me to neurology. I am grateful to the many medical students at Charing Cross and Westminster Medical School who have acted as guinea pigs in the preparation of the book and to the colleagues who have kindly commented on the text.

In learning to be a clinical neurologist and in writing this book I am indebted to a wide range of textbooks and scientific papers, the most important of which are mentioned in the bibliography.

I have been grateful for the continued patience and understanding of my editor, Dilys Jones.

This book is dedicated to Cherith.

INTRODUCTION

Many medical students think that neurological examination is extremely complicated and difficult.

This is because
- they find it hard to remember what to do
- they are not sure what they are looking for
- they do not know how to describe what they find.

The aim of this book is to provide a simple framework to allow a junior medical student to perform a straightforward neurological examination. It explains what to do and points out common problems and mistakes. This book cannot replace conventional bedside teaching and clinical experience.

When trying to simplify the range of neurological findings and their interpretation inevitably not all possible situations can be anticipated. This book has been designed to try and accommodate most common situations and tries to warn of common pitfalls; there will be some occasions where incorrect conclusions will be reached.

How to use this book

This book concentrates on how to perform the neurological part of a physical examination. Each section starts with a brief background with relevant information. This is followed by a section telling you 'What to do', both in a straightforward case and in the presence of abnormalities. The abnormalities that can be found are then described in the 'What you find' section and finally the 'What it means' section provides an interpretation of the findings and suggests potential pathologies.

It is important to understand that the neurological examination can be used as:
- a screening test
- an investigative tool.

It is used as a screening test when you examine a patient in whom you expect to find no neurological abnormalities, for example a patient with a non-neurological disease or a patient with a neurological illness not normally associated with physical abnormalities, for example migraine or epilepsy. Neurological examination is used as an investigative tool in patients where a neurological abnormality is found on screening, or where an abnormality can be expected from the history. The aim of examination is to determine whether there is an abnormality, determining its nature and extent and seeking associated abnormalities.

There is no ideal neurological examination technique. The methods of neurological examination have evolved gradually. There are conventional ways to perform an examination, a conventional order of examination and conventional ways to elicit particular signs. Most neurologists have developed their own system for examination, a variation on the conventional techniques. In this book one such variation is presented and aims to provide a skeleton for students to flesh out with their own personal variations.

In this book each part of the examination is dealt with separately. This is to allow description and understanding of abnormalities in each part of the examination. However these parts need to be considered together in evaluating a patient as a whole. Thus the findings in total need to be synthesised.

The synthesis of the examination findings should be:

1. Anatomical
Can the findings be explained by
- one lesion
- multiple lesions
- a diffuse process?

What level/levels of the nervous systems is/are affected (Fig 0.1)?

2. Syndromal
Do the clinical findings combine to form a recognisable clinical syndrome?

e.g. parkinsonism, motor neurone disease, multiple sclerosis

3. Aetiological
What pathological processes could be consistent with the physical findings?
- genetic
- congenital
- infection
- inflammatory
- neoplastic
- degenerative
- metabolic
- endocrine
- vascular

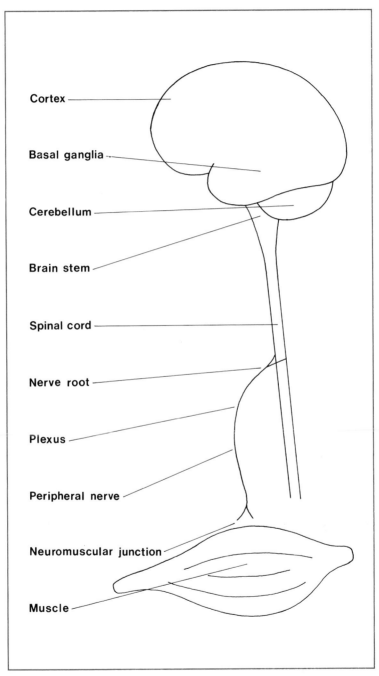

Figure 0.1
The levels of the nervous system

The interpretation of the neurological history and the synthesis of the neurological examination require considerable experience and background knowledge. This book will not be able to provide this. However, using this book you should be able to describe, using appropriate terms, most common neurological abnormalities and begin to synthesise and interpret them.

Throughout the book the patient and examiner are presumed to be male, to avoid the awkward use of he/she.

Cranial nerves will be referred to by their name, or number in roman numerals.

Neurological terms

Neurological terms have evolved and some terms may be used in different ways by different neurologists.

Here are some terms used to describe pathologies at different levels of the nervous system.

-opathy: suffix indicating abnormality at the level of the nervous system indicated in the prefix, see encephalopathy below. Cf **-itis**.

-itis: suffix indicating inflammation of the level of the nervous system indicated in the prefix, see **myelitis** below.

Encephalopathy: abnormality of the brain—may be refined by adjectives such as focal or diffuse, or metabolic or toxic.

Encephalitis: inflammation of the brain. May be refined by adjectives such as focal or diffuse: may be combined with other terms to indicate associated disease—e.g. meningo-encephalitis = meningitis and encephalitis.

Meningitis: inflammation of the meninges.

Myelopathy: abnormality of the spinal cord. Refined by terms indicating aetiology—e.g. radiation, compressive.

Myelitis: inflammation of the spinal cord.

Radiculopathy: abnormality of a nerve root.

Plexopathy: abnormality of nerve plexus (brachial or lumbar).

Peripheral neuropathy: abnormality of peripheral nerves. Usually refined using adjectives such as diffuse/multifocal, sensory/sensorimotor/motor and acute/chronic.

Polyradiculopathy: abnormality of many nerve roots. Usually reserved for proximal nerve damage and to contrast this with length-dependent nerve damage.

Polyneuropathy: similar term to peripheral neuropathy, but may be used to contrast with polyradiculopathy.

Mononeuropathy: abnormality of single nerve.

Myopathy: abnormality of muscle.

Myositis: inflammatory disorder of muscle.

Functional: term used in two ways: 1) non-structural pathology—an abnormality of function, for example migraine; 2) as a term for psychiatrically induced neurological abnormalities including, for example, hysterical conversion.

HISTORY AND EXAMINATION

HISTORY

The history is the most important part of the neurological evaluation. Just as detectives gain most information about the identity of a criminal from witnesses rather than the examination of the scene of the crime, neurologists learn most about the likely pathology from the history rather than the examination.

The general approach to the history is common to all complaints. Which parts of the history will be most important will obviously vary according to the particular complaint. An outline for approaching the history is given below.

When a patient cannot report all events himself or cannot give a history adequately for another reason such as a speech problem it is essential to get the history from others if at all possible, such as relatives, friends or even passers-by.

Determine:

- *The nature of the complaint:* Make sure you understand what the patient is complaining of. For example, dizziness may mean vertigo (the true sensation of spinning) or a swimminess in the head. When a patient says his vision is blurred he may mean it is double. A patient with weakness with no altered sensation may refer to his limb as numb.
- *The extent of any deficit:* For example, what did his weakness prevent him from doing? Was he able to walk normally, did he have to use a stick, could he lift his arm above his head?
- *The onset:* How did it begin? Suddenly, over a few seconds, over a few minutes, hours or days?
- *The time course:* Has it progressed (gradually or in a stepwise fashion), has it progressed and then stabilised, or has it returned intermittently? Again, in describing the progression use a functional gauge where possible, for example the ability to run, walk, using one stick, walking with a frame.

- *The pattern:* If intermittent, what was its duration and what was its frequency?
  Hint: it is better to get an exact description for each event, particularly the first event, rather than an abstracted summary of a typical event.

Also determine:

- *Precipitating or relieving factors*
- *Previous treatments and investigations*
- *Other neurological symptoms.* Determine whether the patient has had any headaches, fits, faints, blackouts, episodes of numbness or tingling or weakness, any sphincter disturbance (urinary or faecal incontinence, urinary retention and constipation) or visual symptoms, including double vision, blurred vision or loss of sight.
- *The current neurological state.* What can the patient do now? Determine current abilities in relation to normal everyday activities. Clearly this needs to be done differently for different types of problem we consider in relation to his work and mobility (can he walk normally or what level of impairment), his ability to eat, wash, go to the toilet.

Common mistakes

Patients frequently want to tell you about the doctors they have seen before, what these doctors have done and said rather than describe what has happened to the patients themselves. This is usually misleading and must be regarded with caution. If this information would be useful to you it is better obtained directly from the doctors concerned. Most patients can be redirected to give their history rather than the history of their medical contacts.

Past medical history

This is clearly important in possibly providing aetiology or associations with neurological conditions. For example, a history of hypertension is important in patients with strokes; diabetes in patients with peripheral neuropathy; previous cancer surgery in patients with focal cerebral abnormalities suggesting possible metastases.

Social history

In neurological patients there may frequently be a significant handicap. In these patients the environment in which they normally live, their financial circumstances, their family and carers in the community are all very important to their current and future care.

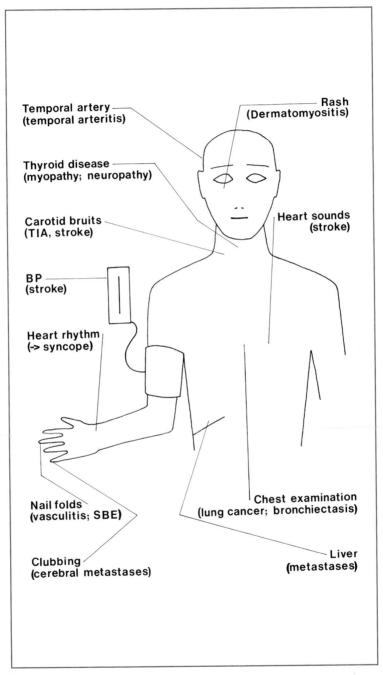

Figure 1.1
General examination of neurological relevance

Toxin exposure

It is important to establish any exposure to toxins including in this category both tobacco and alcohol, as well as industrial neurotoxins.

Systemic inquiry

Systemic inquiry may reveal clues that general medical disease may be presenting with neurological manifestations. For example, a patient with atherosclerosis may have angina and intermittent claudication as well as symptoms of cerebrovascular disease.

GENERAL EXAMINATION

General examination may yield important clues as to the diagnosis of neurological disease. Examination may find systemic disease with neurological complications (Fig. 1.1).

Here are a few examples

Disease	Sign	Neurological condition
Degenerative diseases		
Atherosclerosis	Carotid bruit	Stroke
Valvular heart disease	Murmur	Stroke
Inflammatory disease		
Rheumatoid arthritis	Arthritis and rheumatoid nodules	Neuropathies
Endocrine disease		
Hypothyroidism	Abnormal facies, skin, hair	Cerebellar syndrome, myopathy
Diabetes	Retinal changes Injection marks	Neuropathy
Neoplasia		
Lung cancer	Pleural effusion	Cerebral metastases
Breast cancer	Breast mass	Cerebral metastases
Dermatological disease		
Dermatomyositis	Heliotrope rash	Dermatomyositis

A full general examination is therefore important in assessing a patient with neurological disease. The features that need to be particularly looked for in an unconscious patient are dealt with in section 27.

2

SPEECH

BACKGROUND

Abnormalities of speech need to be considered first as these may interfere with your history-taking and subsequent ability to assess higher function and perform the rest of the examination.

Abnormalities of speech can reflect abnormalities anywhere along the following chain.

Process		Abnormalities
Hearing ↓	———————————	Deafness
Understanding ↓ Thought and word finding ↓	} ———————————	Aphasia
Voice production ↓	———————————	Dysphonia
Articulation	———————————	Dysarthria

Problems with deafness are dealt with in section 12.

1. Aphasia

In this book the term aphasia will be used to refer to all disorders of understanding, thought and word finding. Dysphasia is a term used by some to indicate a disorder of speech reserving aphasia to mean absence of speech.

Aphasia has been classified in a number of ways and each new classification has brought some new terminology. There are therefore a number of terms that refer to broadly similar problems:

Synonyms

Broca's aphasia = expressive aphasia = motor aphasia
Wernicke's aphasia = receptive aphasia = sensory aphasia
nominal aphasia = anomic aphasia

Most of these systems have evolved from a simple model of aphasia (Fig. 2.1).

In this model sounds are recognised as language in Wernicke's area, which is then connected to a 'concept area' where the meaning of the words are understood. The 'concept area' is connected to Broca's area where speech output is generated. Wernicke's area is also connected directly to Broca's area by the arcuate fasciculus. These areas are in the dominant hemisphere and are described later. The left hemisphere is dominant in right-handed patients and some left-handed patients, and the right hemisphere is dominant in some left-handed patients.

The following patterns of aphasia can be recognised associated with lesions at the sites as numbered:

1. **Wernicke's aphasia** — poor comprehension, fluent but often meaningless (as it cannot be internally checked) speech. No repetition.

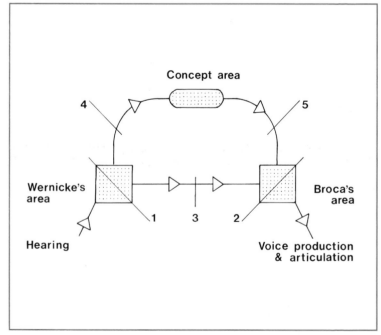

Figure 2.1
Simple model of speech understanding and output

2. **Broca's aphasia** — preserved comprehension, non-fluent speech. No repetition.
3. **Conductive aphasia** — loss of repetition with preserved comprehension and output.
4. **Transcortical sensory aphasia** — as in (1) but with preserved repetition.
5. **Transcortical motor aphasia** — as in (2) but with preserved repetition.

Reading and writing are further aspects of language. These can also be included in models such as the one above. Not surprisingly the models become quite complicated!

2. Dysphonia

This is a disturbance of voice production and may reflect either local vocal cord pathology (such as laryngitis), an abnormality of the nerve supply via the vagus or occasionally a psychological disturbance.

3. Dysarthria

Voice production requires coordination of breathing, vocal cords, larynx, palate, tongue and lips. Dysarthria can therefore reflect difficulties at different levels.

Lesions of upper motor neurone type, of the extrapyramidal system (such as Parkinson's disease) and cerebellar lesions disturb the integration of processes of speech production and tend to disturb the rhythm of speech.

Lesions of one or several of the cranial nerves tend to produce characteristic distortion of certain parts of speech.

1. APHASIA

WHAT TO DO

Speech abnormalities may hinder or prevent taking a history from the patient. If so, **take history from relatives or friends**.

Establish if **right- or left-handed**.

Discover his **first language**.

Assess understanding

Ask the patient a simple question
- what is your name and address?
- what is/was your job? Explain exactly what you do
- where do you come from?

If he does not appear to understand:
Repeat louder

Test his understanding

- Ask questions with **yes/no answers**
  e.g. 'Is this a pen?' (showing something else, then a pen)
- Give a **simple command**
  e.g. 'Open your mouth' or 'With your right hand touch your nose'
  If successful:
  - try more **complicated commands**
    e.g. 'With your right hand touch your nose and then your left ear'

  Remember if weak he may not be able to perform the simple tasks. Define how much is understood.

Assess spontaneous speech

If he does appear to understand but is unable to speak:

- Ask if he has difficulty in finding the right words
  This often brings a nod and a smile indicating pleasure that you understand the problem
- If less severe he may be able to tell you his name and address slowly

  - **Ask further questions**
    e.g. about his job or how his problem started
    Is speech fluent? Does he use words correctly?
    Does he use the wrong word—*paraphasia*—or is it **meaning-less jargon** (sometimes called *jargon aphasia*)?

Assess word finding ability and naming

- Ask him to name all the animals he can think of (*normal* 18–22 in 1 minute)
- Ask him to give all the words beginning with a particular letter, usually 'f' or 's' (*abnormal* < 12 in 1 minute for each letter)

These are tests of word finding. This test can be quantified by counting the number of objects within a standard time.

- Ask him to name familiar objects that are to hand, e.g. a watch, watch strap, buckle, shirt, tie, buttons
  Start with easily named objects and later ask about less frequently used objects that will be more difficult.

Assess repetition

- Ask the patient to repeat a simple phrase, e.g. 'the sun is shining', and then increasingly complicated phrases

Assess severity of impairment of speech

- Is the aphasia **socially incapacitating**?

FURTHER TESTS

Test reading and writing

Check there is no visual impairment and that usual reading glasses are used.

Ask the patient to:
- read a sentence
- obey written command — e.g. 'close your eyes'
- write a sentence (check there is no motor disability to prevent this)

Impaired reading = *dyslexia*, impaired writing = *dysgraphia*

WHAT YOU FIND

See Flow Chart 1.

Before continuing your examination **describe your findings** — e.g. 'This man has a socially incapacitating non-fluent global aphasia which is predominantly expressive, with paraphasia and impaired repetition. There is associated dyslexia and dysgraphia.'

WHAT IT MEANS

- ○ **Aphasia**: Lesion in the *dominant* (usually left) hemisphere
- ○ **Global aphasia**: Lesion in *dominant* hemisphere affecting both *Wernicke's* and *Broca's* areas (Fig. 2.2)
- ○ **Wernicke's aphasia**: Lesion in *Wernicke's* area (supramarginal gyrus of the parietal lobe and upper part of temporal lobe). May be associated with *field defect*
- ○ **Broca's aphasia**: Lesion in *Broca's* area (inferior frontal gyrus). May be associated with a *hemiplegia*
- ○ **Conductive aphasia**: Lesion in arcuate fasciculus
- ○ **Transcortical sensory aphasia**: Lesion in posterior parieto-occipital region
- ○ **Transcortical motor aphasia**: Incomplete lesion in Broca's area
- ○ **Nominal aphasia**: Lesion in *angular gyrus*
- ○ Common causes are given on p. 35.

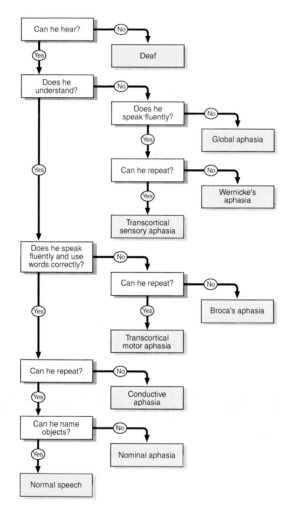

Flow chart 1
Aphasia

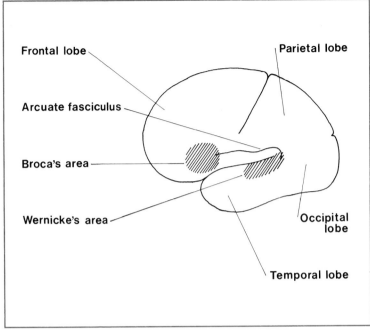

Figure 2.2
Diagram of the brain showing the location of Broca's and Wernicke's area

2. DYSPHONIA

WHAT TO DO
If the patient is able to give his name and address but is unable to produce normal volume of sound or speaks in a whisper this is *dysphonia*.
- **Ask the patient to cough.** Listen to the quality of the cough
- **Ask the patient to say a sustained 'eeeeee'.** Does it fatigue?

WHAT YOU FIND AND WHAT IT MEANS

○ normal cough — the motor supply to the vocal cords is intact
○ dysphonia + normal cough — local laryngeal problems or hysteria
○ cough lacks explosive start: a bovine cough — vocal cord palsy
○ the note cannot be sustained, and fatigues — consider myasthenia

3. DYSARTHRIA

WHAT TO DO

If the patient is able to give his name and address but the words are not formed properly, he has dysarthria (see Flow Chart 2).

- **Ask him to repeat difficult phrases** — e.g. Peter Piper picked a peck of pickled pepper, the Leith policeman dismisseth us
  Two very useful phrases are
  - 'yellow lorry' — tests lingual (tongue) sounds
  - 'baby hippopotamus' — tests labial (lip) sounds.

  Listen carefully for:
  - the rhythm of the speech
  - are the words slurred?
  - which sounds cause the greatest difficulty

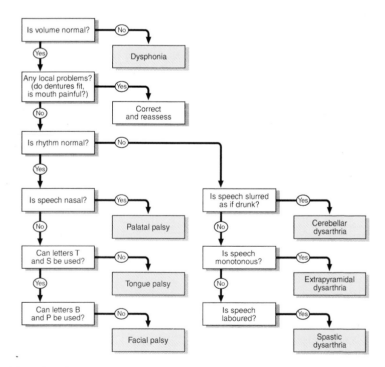

Flow chart 2
Dysarthria

WHAT YOU FIND

Types of dysarthria

- ○ **Spastic**: slurred, patient hardly opens mouth, as if trying to speak from the back of mouth
- ○ **Extrapyramidal**: monotonous, without rhythm, sentences suddenly start and stop
- ○ **Cerebellar**: slurred as if drunk, disjointed rhythm sometimes with scanning speech (equal emphasis on each syllable)
- ○ **Lower motor neurone**:
    - – *palatal*: nasal speech, as with a bad cold
    - – *tongue*: distorted speech, especially letters t, s, d
    - – *facial*: difficulty with b, p, m, w, the sounds avoided by ventriloquists
- ○ **Myasthenic**: Muscle fatiguability demonstrated by making patient count. Observe for development of dysphonia or lower motor neurone pattern of dysarthria. (N.B. Myasthenia gravis is a failure of neuromuscular transmission.)

Before continuing your examination **describe your findings**.

WHAT IT MEANS

- ○ **Spastic dysarthria**: bilateral upper motor neurone weakness— *causes*: pseudobulbar palsy, motor neurone disease
- ○ **Extrapyramidal dysarthria**—*common cause*: parkinsonism
- ○ **Cerebellar dysarthria**—*common causes*: alcohol intoxication, multiple sclerosis, phenytoin toxicity; *rarely*: hereditary ataxias
- ○ **Lower motor neurone dysarthria**—*causes*: lesions of X (palatal), XII (tongue) or VII (facial): see relevant sections

3

MENTAL STATE AND HIGHER FUNCTION

1. MENTAL STATE

BACKGROUND

In this section examination of higher function has been separated from examination of mental state. This is because higher function can be examined using relatively simple tests while mental state is examined using observation of the patient and attention to points within the history.

Mental state

The mental state relates to the mood and thoughts of a patient. Abnormalities may reflect:
- **neurological disease**, such as frontal lobe disease or dementia
- **psychiatric illness** which may be causing neurological symptoms (e.g. anxiety leading to panic attacks)
- **psychiatric illness secondary to neurological disease** (e.g. depression following stroke).

Mental state examination attempts to distinguish:
- **focal neurological deficit**
- **diffuse neurological deficit**
- **primary psychiatric illness** such as depression, anxiety or hysteria presenting with somatic symptoms
- **psychiatric illness** secondary to, or associated with neurological disease.

Mental state examination is likely to be normal in most patients who therefore need only the simplest assessment. However it pays to consider whether further evaluation is needed in all patients.

Methods of formal psychiatric assessment will not be dealt with here.

WHAT TO DO AND WHAT YOU FIND

Appearance and behaviour

Watch the patient while you take the history. Here are some questions you can ask yourself in assessing the appearance and behaviour.

Are there signs of self-neglect?
- dirty or unkempt — consider *depression, dementia, alcoholism* or *drug abuse*

Does the patient appear depressed?
- furrowed brow, immobile, downcast facies, slow monotonous speech (cf parkinsonism, section 24)

Does the patient appear anxious?
- fidgety, restless

Does the patient behave appropriately?
- overfamiliar and disinhibited or aggressive — consider *frontalism*
- unresponsive, with little emotional response — *flat affect*

Does the patient's mood change rapidly?
- crying or laughing easily — *emotional lability*

Does the patient show appropriate concern about his symptoms and disability?
- lack of concern in the face of significant disability ('belle indifference') — consider *hysterical disease*

Mood

Ask the patient about his mood
- how are your spirits at the moment?
- how would you describe your mood?

If you consider the patient may be depressed, ask:
- are you ever able to cheer up?
- do you see any hope in the future?

Patients with depression say they find it difficult to cheer up and see little hope in the future.

Patients with schizophrenia often have an apparent lack of mood — *blunted affect* — or inappropriate mood, smiling when you expect him to be sad — *incongruous affect*.

In mania, patients are euphoric.

Vegetative symptoms

Ask the patient about vegetative symptoms

- weight loss or gain
- sleep disturbance (waking early or difficulty getting to sleep)
- appetite
- constipation
- libido

Look for symptoms of anxiety

- palpitation
- sweating
- hyperventilation (tingling in fingers, toes and around the mouth, dry mouth, dizziness, and often a feeling of breathlessness)

Delusions

A delusion is a firmly held belief, not altered by rational argument, and not a conventional belief within the culture and society of the patient.

Delusional ideas may be revealed in the history but cannot be elicited by direct questioning. They can be classified according to their form (e.g. persecutory, grandiose, hypochondriacal) as well as by describing their content.

Delusions are seen in acute confusional states and psychotic illnesses.

Hallucinations and illusions

When a patient complains that he has seen, heard, felt or smelt something, you must decide whether it is an illusion or a hallucination.

An **illusion** is a misinterpretation of external stimuli and it is particularly common in patients with altered consciousness. For example, a confused patient says he can see a giant fist shaking outside the window, which is in fact a tree blowing in the wind outside.

A **hallucination** is a perception experienced without external stimuli that is indistinguishable from the perception of a real external stimulus.

Hallucinations may be *elementary*—flashes of light, bangs whistles—or *complex*—seeing people, faces, hearing voices or music. Elementary hallucinations are usually organic.

Hallucinations can be described according to the type of sensation:

- *smell* — olfactory ⎫
- *taste* — gustatory ⎬ usually organic
- *sight* — visual ⎭
- *touch* — somatic ⎫
- *hearing* — auditory ⎬ usually psychiatric

Before continuing **describe your findings**, e.g. 'An elderly unkempt man, who responds slowly but appropriately to questions and appears depressed.'

WHAT IT MEANS

In psychiatric diagnoses there is a hierarchy, and the psychiatric diagnosis is taken from the highest level involved. For example a patient with both anxiety (low-level symptom) and psychotic symptoms (higher-level symptom) would be considered to have a psychosis.

```
Highest
   Organic psychoses
   Functional psychoses  — schizophrenia
                         — psychotic depression
                         — bipolar (manic) depression
   Neuroses              — depression
                         — anxiety states
                         — hysterical reaction
                         — phobias
                         — obsessional neurosis
   Personality disorders
Lowest
```

Organic psychosis

A neurological deficit producing an altered mental state — suggested by: altered consciousness, fluctuating level of consciousness, disturbed memory, visual, olfactory, somatic and gustatory hallucinations and sphincter disturbance.

Proceed to test higher function for localising signs.
Three major syndromes:

○ **Acute confusional state** — *common causes*: drug induced, (especially sedative drugs, including antidepressants and antipsychotics), metabolic disturbances (especially hypoglycaemia), alcohol withdrawal, seizure related (post ictal or temporal lobe seizures)

○ **Dysmnesic syndromes** — prominent loss of short term memory e.g. Korsakoff's psychosis (thiamine deficiency)

○ **Dementia** — *common causes* given after higher function testing

Functional psychoses

- **Schizophrenia**: clear consciousness, flat or incongruous affect, concrete thinking (see below), prominent delusions, formed auditory hallucinations, usually voices, which may speak to or about him. May feel he is being controlled. May adopt strange postures and stay in them (catatonia)
- **Psychotic depression**: clear consciousness, depressed affect, no longer self-caring, slow, reports delusions (usually self-deprecating) or hallucinations. Usually vegetative symptoms — early waking, weight loss, reduced appetite, loss of libido, constipation
  N.B.: considerable overlap with neurotic depression
- **Bipolar depression**: episodes of depression as above, but also episodes of mania — elevated mood, grandiose delusions, pressure of speech and thought

Neuroses

- **Depression**: low mood, loss of energy — following an identifiable event (e.g. bereavement). Vegetative symptoms less prominent
- **Anxiety state**: debilitating anxiety without reasonable cause, prone to panic attacks, may hyperventilate
- **Hysterical reaction**: unconscious production or increase of a disability, associated with an inappropriate reaction to disability. There may be a secondary gain. Disability often does not conform to anatomical patterns of neurological loss
- **Phobias**: irrational fear of something — ranging from open space to spiders
- **Obsessional states**: a thought repeatedly intrudes into the patient's consciousness, often forcing him to actions (compulsions) — e.g. thought that patient is contaminated forces him to repeatedly wash his hands. Patients may develop rituals

Personality disorder

Lifelong extreme form of normal range of personalities. For example:
- lacking ability to form relationships, abnormally aggressive and irresponsible = *psychopathic personality*
- histrionic, deceptive, immature = *hysterical personality*

2. HIGHER FUNCTION

BACKGROUND

Higher function is a term used to encompass thought, memory understanding, perception and intellect.

There are many sophisticated tests of higher function. These can be applied to test intelligence as well as in disease. However, much can be learned from simple bedside testing.

The purpose of testing is to:
- document the level of function in a reproducible way
- distinguish focal and diffuse deficits
- assess functional level within the community.

Higher function can be divided into the following parts:
- attention
- memory (immediate short-term and long-term)
- calculation
- abstract thought
- spatial
- visual and body perception.

All testing relies on intact speech. This should be tested first. The tests cannot be interpreted if the patient has poor attention as clearly this will interfere with all other aspects of testing. Results need to be interpreted in the light of premorbid intelligence. For example, the significance of an error in calculation clearly differs when found in a labourer and in a professor of mathematics.

A mini mental state test (MMS) given on p. 25 is a simple, easily-applied test which gives a score out of 30. It is a useful guide for documenting the level of function repeatedly but not for distinguishing focal from diffuse loss.

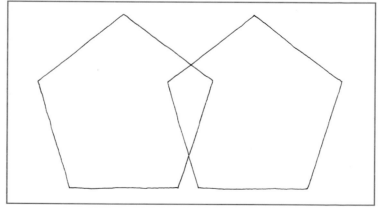

Figure 3.1
Pair of intersecting pentagons for mini mental state test

Mini mental state test

Orientation

Score one point for correct answers to each of the following questions:

What is the: time? date? day? month? year?   (5 points)

What is the name of this: ward? hospital? district? town? country?
                                                    (5 points)

Registration

Name three objects. Score up to 3 points if, at the first attempt, the patient repeats, in order, the three objects you have randomly named. Score 2 or one if this is the number he repeats correctly. Endeavour, by further attempts and prompting, to have all three repeated, so as to test recall later.   (3 points)

Attention and calculation

Ask the patient to subtract 7 from 100, and then 7 from the result — repeat this five times, scoring one for each time a correct subtraction is performed.   (5 points)

Recall

Ask for the three objects repeated in the registration test, scoring one for each correctly recalled.   (3 points)

Language

Score one point for two objects (a pencil and a watch) correctly named.
                                                    (2 points)

Score one point if the following phrase is correctly repeated 'No ifs, ands or buts'.   (1 point)

Score 3 if a three-stage command is correctly executed; score 1 for each stage: for example, 'with the index finger of your right hand touch the tip of your nose and then your left ear,' or 'take this piece of paper in your right hand, fold it in half and place it on the floor.'   (3 points)

On a blank piece of paper write, 'Close your eyes' and ask the patient to obey what is written. Score one point if he closes his eyes.   (1 point)

Ask the patient to write a sentence. Score one if the sentence is sensible and has a verb and a subject.   (1 point)

Construct a pair of intersecting pentagons, each side 1 inch long (Fig. 3.1). Score one if this is correctly copied.   (1 point)

TOTAL	30points

What it means

Less than 23 = *cognitively impaired*

N.B. Does not distinguish focal from diffuse disease. Aphasic patients do especially badly.

Apraxia is a term used to describe an inability to perform a task when there is no weakness or inco-ordination or movement disorder to prevent it. It will be described here though clearly requires examination of the motor system before it can be assessed.

WHEN TO TEST HIGHER FUNCTION?

When should you test higher function formally? Obviously if the patient complains of loss of memory or of any alteration in higher function you should proceed. In other patients the clues that should lead you to test come from the history. Patients are often adept at covering their loss of memory: vague answers to specific questions, inconsistencies given without apparent concern — may suggest the need for testing. If in doubt, test. History from the relatives and friends is essential.

When you test higher function the tests should be applied as:
1. an investigative tool directed towards the problem
2. screening tests to look for evidence of involvement of other higher functions.

For example, if a patient complains of poor memory the examiner should test attention, short-term memory and longer-term memory and then screen for involvement of calculation, abstract thought and spatial orientation.

WHAT TO DO

Introduction

Before starting, explain that you are going to ask a number of questions. Apologise that some of these questions may seem very simple.

Test attention, orientation, memory and calculation whenever you test higher function (often best done with MMS test). The other tests should be applied more selectively, indications will be outlined.

1. Attention and orientation

Orientation: test orientation in time, place and person
- *time*: What day is it? What is the date? What is the month, the year? What is the season? What is the time of day?
- *place*: What is the name of the place we are in? What is the name of the ward/hospital? What is the name of the town/city?
- *person*: What is your name? What is your job? Where do you live?

Make a note of errors made

Attention: Digit span
Tell the patient that you want him to repeat some numbers that you give him. Start with three- or four-digit numbers and increase until the patient makes several mistakes at one number of digits. Then explain that you want him to repeat the numbers backwards, for example: 'When I say one, two, three you say three, two, one.'

Note the number of digits the patient is able to recall forwards and backwards.

- *normal*: seven forward, five backwards

Hint: use parts of telephone numbers you know (not 999)

2. Memory

a. Immediate recall and attention
Name and address test
Tell the patient that you want him to remember a name and address, and give the patient a three-line name and address, e.g. John Brown, 5 Rose Cottages, Ruislip. Ask him immediately to repeat it back to you.

Note how many errors are made in repeating it and how many times you have to repeat it before it is repeated correctly.

- *normal*: immediate registration

Hint: develop a name and address that you use regularly so you don't make mistakes yourself.

Alternative test:
Babcock sentence
Ask the patient to repeat this sentence: 'One thing a nation must have to be rich and great is a large, secure supply of wood.'

- *normal*: correct in three attempts

b. Short-term memory
About 5 minutes after asking the patient to remember the name and address ask him to repeat it.

Note how many mistakes are made.
Hint: the 5 minutes can be spent testing calculation and abstract thought.

c. Long-term memory

Test factual knowledge you would expect the patient to have. This varies greatly from patient to patient and you need to tailor it accordingly. For example, a retired soldier should know the commander-in-chief in the Second World War, a football fan the year England won the World Cup, a neurologist the names of the cranial nerves. The following may be used as examples of general knowledge: dates of the Second World War, the American president who was shot dead.

3. Calculation

Serial sevens

Ask the patient if he is good with numbers, explaining that you are going to ask him to do some simple calculations. Ask him to take seven from a hundred, then seven from what remains.

Note mistakes and the time taken to perform calculation.

Alternative test — especially if serial sevens prove too difficult:
  Doubling threes
  This should be used if the patient professes difficulty with calculations. What is two times three? Twice that? And keep on doubling.

  Note how high the patient is able to go and how long it takes.

Further tests:
Ask the patient to perform increasingly difficult mental arithmetic: $2 + 3$; $7 + 12$; $21 - 9$; 4×7; $36 \div 9$; etc.
N.B. adjust to premorbid expectations.

4. Abstract thought

This tests for frontal lobe function: useful with frontal lobe lesions, dementia and psychiatric illness.
Tell the patient that you would like him to explain some proverbs for you.

Ask him to explain well-known proverbs. For example: 'A rolling stone gathers no moss,' 'People in glass houses shouldn't throw stones,' 'A stitch in time saves nine.'

Does he give the correct interpretation?

What you find
○ Correct interpretation: *normal*
○ Physical interpretation: for example, the stone just rolls down so moss doesn't stick, or throwing stones will break the glass. This indicates *concrete thinking*.

Ask him to explain the difference between pairs of objects
    e.g. a skirt and a pair of trousers, a table and a chair

Ask the patient to estimate: the number of people in England and Wales (49 million); the length of a jumbo jet (70 m or 230 feet); the weight of an elephant (5 tonnes); the height of the Eiffel tower (986 feet or 300 m)

What you find
○ Reasonable estimates — *normal*
○ Unreasonable estimates — indicates *abnormal abstract thinking.*

5. Spatial

This tests for parietal and occipital lobe function. Also useful in dementias.

Clock face
Ask the patient to draw a clock face and to fill in the numbers. Ask him then to draw the hands on at a given time, for example ten to four.

Map test
Ask the patient to indicate the site of cities on a map outline (Fig. 3.2).

Five-pointed star
Ask the patient to copy a five-pointed star (Fig. 3.3).

What you find
○ Accurate clock and star: *normal*
○ Half clock missing: *visual inattention*
○ Unable to draw clock or reproduce star: *constructional apraxia.*
N.B. This is difficult to assess in the presence of weakness.

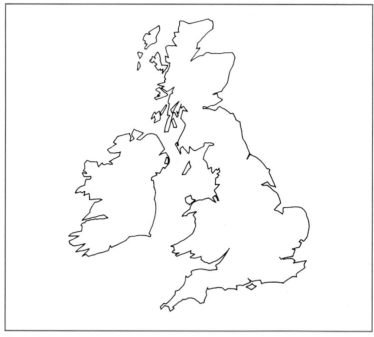

Figure 3.2
Map outline — where is Birmingham?

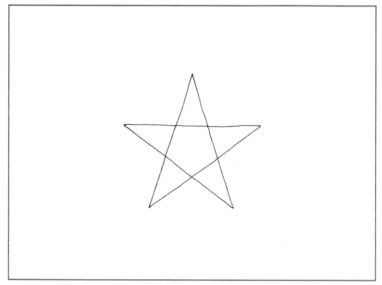

Figure 3.3
Five-pointed star

6. Visual and body perception

Test for parietal and occipital lesions. Useful in dementias.

Abnormalities of perception of sensation despite normal sensory pathways are called *agnosias*. Agnosias can occur in all types of sensation but clinically usually affect vision, touch and body perception.

The sensory pathway needs to have been examined and found to be intact before considering a patients has an agnosia. However agnosia is usually considered as part of higher function and is therefore considered here.

Facial recognition: 'famous faces'

Take bedside newspaper or magazine and ask the patient to identify the faces of famous people. Choose people the patient will be expected to know: the Queen, the Prime Minister, and so on.

Note mistakes made.
- Recognises faces: *normal*
- Does not recognise faces: *prosopagnosia*

Body perception:

- Patient ignores one side (usually left) and is unable to find hand if asked (*hemi-neglect*)
- Patient does not recognise left hand if shown it (*asomatagnosia*)
- Patient is unaware of weakness of affected (usually left) side — *anosagnosia* — and will often move the right side when asked to move the left

Ask the patient to show you his index finger, ring finger and so on
- failure — *finger agnosia*

Ask the patient to touch his right ear with his left index finger. Cross your hands and ask which is your right hand
- failure — *left/right agnosia*

Sensory agnosia

Ask the patient to close his eyes and place an object — e.g. coin, key, paperclip — in his hand and ask him what it is.
- failure — *astereognosis*

Ask the patient to close his eyes and write a number or letter on his hand and ask him what it is.
- failure — *agraphaesthesia*.
  Hint: test on the unaffected side first to ensure patient understands the test.

7. Apraxia

Tests for parietal lobe and premotor cortex of the frontal lobe function; very useful in dementias.

Ask the patient to perform an imaginary task: 'Show me how you would comb your hair, drink a cup of tea, strike a match and blow it out'.

Observe the patient. *If there is a difficulty* give the patient an appropriate object and see if he is able to do it with the appropriate prompt. *If there is further difficulty* demonstrate and ask him to copy what you are doing.

- The patient is able to perform the act appropriately — *normal*
- The patient is unable to initiate the action though understanding the command — *ideational apraxia*
- The patient performs the task but makes errors, for example uses his hand as a cup rather than an imaginary cup — *ideomotor apraxia*

If inability is related to a specific task, for example dressing, this should be referred to as a *dressing apraxia*. This is often tested in hospital by asking the patient to put on a dressing gown with one sleeve pulled inside out. The patient should normally be able to overcome this easily.

Three hand test

Ask the patient to copy your hand movements and demonstrate: 1) make a fist and tap it on the table with your thumb upwards; 2) then straighten out your fingers and tap on the table with your thumb upwards; 3) then place your palm flat on the table. *If the patient is unable to perform this after one demonstration*, repeat the demonstration.

- if the patient is unable to perform this in the presence of normal motor function — *limb apraxia*

What you find

Three patterns can be recognised:

1. Patients with poor attention
Tests useful to document level of function, but are of limited use in distinguishing focal from diffuse disease. Assess as in section 27.

2. Patients with deficits in many or all major areas of testing
Indicates a diffuse or multifocal process.
If of slow onset — *dementia* or *chronic brain syndrome*
If of more rapid onset — *confusional state* or *acute brain syndrome*.

Common mistakes
Dementia needs to be distinguished from:
- ○ **low intelligence** — usually indicated from a history of intellectual attainment

○ **depression**—may be difficult especially in the elderly. Often suggested by the patient's demeanour

○ **aphasia**—usually found on critical testing

3. Patients with deficits in one or only a few areas of testing

Indicates focal process. Identify area affected and seek associated physical signs (see Patterns of focal loss).

Patterns of focal loss

Lobe	Alteration in higher function	Associations
Frontal	Apathy, disinhibition	Contralateral hemiplegia, Broca's aphasia (dominant hemisphere), primitive reflexes
Temporal	Memory	Wernicke's aphasia (dominant hemisphere), upper quadrantanopia
Parietal	Calculation, perceptual and spatial orientation (non-dominant hemisphere)	Apraxia (dominant hemisphere) Homonymous hemianopia, hemisensory disturbance, neglect
Occipital	Perceptual and spatial orientation	Hemianopia

1. **Impaired attention and orientation**: occurs with diffuse disturbance of cerebral function

   If *acute* often associated with disturbance of consciousness—assess as section 27

   If *chronic* limits ability for further testing—suggestive of dementia

   N.B. Also occurs with anxiety, depression

2. **Memory**: loss of short-term memory in alert patient—usually bilateral—limbic system (hippocampus, mamillary bodies) disturbance—seen in diffuse encephalopathies; bilateral temporal lesions; prominent in Korsakoff's psychosis (thiamine deficiency). Loss of long-term memory with preserved short-term memory—functional memory loss

3. **Calculation**: impaired calculation usually indicates diffuse encephalopathy. If associated with finger agnosia (inability to name fingers), left–right agnosia (inability to distinguish left from right) and dysgraphia = Gerstmann syndrome—indicates a dominant parietal lobe syndrome.

   Perverse but consistent calculation errors may suggest psychiatric disease.

4. **Abstract thought**

   If interpretations of proverbs are concrete—suggests diffuse encephalopathy.

   If interpretation includes delusional ideas—suggests psychiatric illness, with particular frontal lobe involvement.

   Poor estimates suggest frontal or diffuse encephalopathy or psychiatric illness.

5. **Loss of spatial appreciation** (copying drawings, astereognosis)—parietal lobe lesions.

6. **Visual and body perception**

   Prosopagnosia—bilateral temporo-parietal lesions

   Neglect

   Sensory agnosia ⎫

   Astereognosis ⎬ parietal lobe lesions

   Agraphaesthesiae ⎭

7. **Apraxia**

   Ideomotor apraxia—lesion either of the dominant parietal lobe, premotor cortex or a diffuse brain lesion.

   Ideational apraxia—suggests bilateral parietal disease.

WHAT IT MEANS

Diffuse or multifocal abnormalities

Common

○ Alzheimer's disease

○ Vascular disease (multi-infarct)

Rare

Degenerative conditions:

○ Pick's disease

○ Huntington's disease

Nutritional:

○ Thiamine deficiency (Korsakoff's psychosis)

○ Vitamin B_{12} deficiency

Infective:

○ Quaternary syphilis

○ Creutzfeldt–Jakob disease

○ HIV encephalopathy

Structural:

○ Normal pressure hydrocephalus

○ Demyelination

○ Multiple sclerosis

Focal deficits

May indicate early stage of a multifocal disease

Vascular:
- Thrombosis, emboli or haemorrhage

Neoplastic:
- Primary or secondary tumours

Infective:
- Abscess

Demyelination:
- Multiple sclerosis

4

GAIT

BACKGROUND

Always examine patient's gait. It is a co-ordinated action requiring integration of sensory and motor functions. The gait may be the only abnormality on examination, or it may lead you to seek appropriate clinical associations on the rest of the examination. The most commonly seen are: hemiplegic, parkinsonian, marche à petits pas, ataxic and unsteady gaits.

Romberg's test is conveniently performed after examining the gait. This is a simple test primarily of joint position sense.

WHAT TO DO AND WHAT YOU FIND

Ask the patient to walk

Ensure you are able to see the arms and legs adequately.

Is the gait symmetrical?
- yes: see Flow Chart 3 and Figure 4.1
- no: see below

(Gaits can usually be divided into symmetrical and asymmetrical even though the symmetry is not perfect)

If symmetrical:
Look at the size of paces
- small or normal?

If small paces:
Look at the posture and arm swing
- stooped with reduced armswing — *parkinsonian* (may be difficult to start and stop — *festinant* — may be worse on one side; tremor may be seen to increase on walking)
- upright with marked armswing — *marche à petits pas*

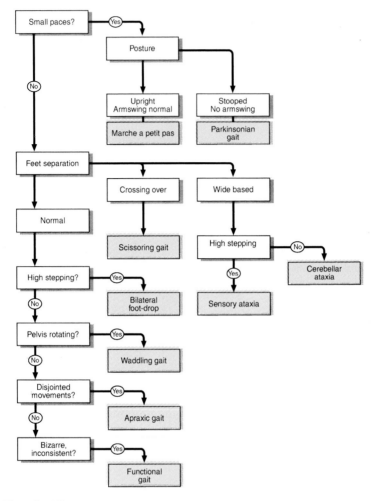

Flow chart 3
Gait

Symmetrical Gaits

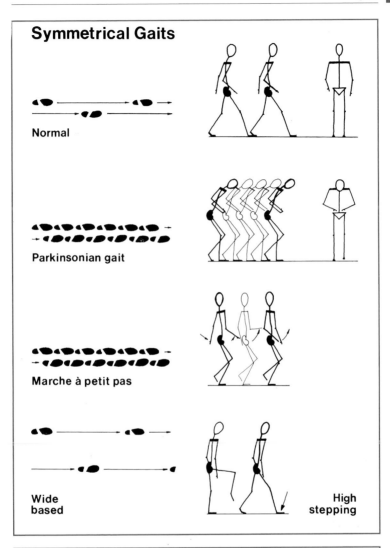

Normal

Parkinsonian gait

Marche à petit pas

Wide based

High stepping

Asymmetrical Gait

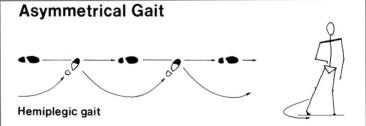

Hemiplegic gait

Figure 4.1

If normal paces:
Look at the lateral distance between the feet
- normal
- widely separated — *broad-based*
- legs unco-ordinated — *cerebellar*
- crossing over, toes dragged — *scissoring*

Look at the knees
- normal
- knees lifted high — *high-stepping*

Look at the pelvis and shoulders
- normal
- marked rotation of pelvis and shoulder — *waddling*

Look at the whole movement
- normal
- disjointed as if forgotten how to walk, patient frequently appears rooted to spot — *apraxic*
- bizarre, elaborate and inconsistent — *functional*

If asymmetrical
Is the patient in pain?
- yes — *painful or antalgic gait*

Look for a bony deformity
- orthopaedic gait

Does one leg swing out to the side?
- yes — *hemiplegic gait*

Look at the knee heights
- normal
- one knee lifts higher — *foot drop*

FURTHER TESTS

Ask the patient to walk as if on a tight-rope *(demonstrate)*
- if patient falls consistently — *unsteady*
- may fall predominantly to one side
- elderly patients are often slightly unsteady.

Ask the patient to walk on his heels *(demonstrate)*
- if unable to — *foot drop*

Ask the patient to walk on his toes *(demonstrate)*
- if unable — *weakness of gastrocnemius*

WHAT IT MEANS

- **Parkinsonian**: indicates basal ganglion dysfunction — *common causes*: Parkinson's disease, major tranquillisers
- **Marche à petits pas**: indicates bilateral diffuse cortical dysfunction — *common causes*: diffuse cerebrovascular disease 'lacunar state'
- **Scissoring**: indicates spastic paraparesis — *common causes*: cerebral palsy, multiple sclerosis, cord compression
- **Sensory ataxia**: indicates loss of joint position sense (Romberg's positive) — *common causes*: peripheral neuropathy, posterior column loss (see below)
- **Cerebellar ataxia**: veers towards side of lesion — *common causes*: drugs (e.g. phenytoin), alcohol, multiple sclerosis, cerebrovascular disease
- **Waddling gait**: indicates weak or ineffective proximal muscles — *common causes*: proximal myopathies, bilateral congenital dislocation of the hip
- **Apraxic gait**: indicates the cortical integration of the movement is abnormal, usually with frontal lobe pathology — *common causes*: normal pressure hydrocephalus, cerebrovascular disease
- **Hemiplegic**: unilateral upper motor neurone lesion — *common causes*: stroke, multiple sclerosis
- **Foot drop**: *common causes* — unilateral: common peroneal palsy, pyramidal lesion, L5 radiculopathy. Bilateral: peripheral neuropathy.
- **Functional gait**: variable, may be inconsistent with rest of examination, worse when watched. May be mistaken for the gait in chorea (especially Huntington's disease), which is shuffling, twitching and spasmodic and has associated findings on examination (see section 24)

Non-neurological gaits

- **Painful gait**: *common causes*: arthritis, trauma — usually obvious.
- **Orthopaedic gait**: *common causes:* shortened limb, previous hip surgery, trauma.

Romberg's test

What to do
Ask the patient to stand with his feet together
- allow him to stand like this for a few seconds

Tell the patient you are ready to catch him if he falls (make sure you are)
- if he falls with his eyes open you cannot proceed with the test

If not:
Ask the patient to close his eyes

What you find and what it means

○ **Stands with eyes open; stands with eyes closed** = Romberg's test is negative — *normal*

○ **Stands with eyes open; falls with eyes closed** = Romberg's test is positive — *loss of joint position sense*

> *This can occur with*
>
> 1. **posterior column lesion in the spinal cord**: *common causes* — cord compression (e.g. cervical spondylosis, tumour); *rarer causes* — tabes dorsalis, vitamin B_{12} deficiency, degenerative spinal cord disease
>
> 2. **peripheral neuropathy**: *common causes* — see section 20

○ **Unable to stand with eyes open and feet together** = severe unsteadiness — *common causes*: cerebellar syndromes and both central and peripheral vestibular syndromes

○ **Stands with eyes open; rocks backwards and forwards with eyes closed** — suggests a cerebellar syndrome.

Common mistakes

• Romberg's test *cannot* be performed if the patients cannot stand unaided

• Romberg's test is *not* positive in cerebellar disease

5

GENERAL

BACKGROUND

Cranial nerve abnormalities may arise (see Fig. 5.1):
a. from specific lesions to the nerve
b. from a lesion in the nucleus
c. in communicating pathways to and from the cortex, diencephalon (thalamus and associated structures), cerebellum or other parts of the brainstem
d. as generalised problems of nerve or muscle.

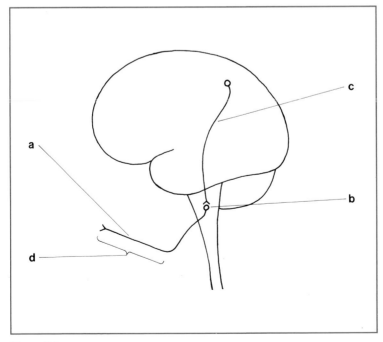

Figure 5.1
Location of cranial nerve abnormalities (see text for key)

When examining the cranial nerves you need to establish whether there is an abnormality, the nature of the abnormality, the extent and any associations.

More than one cranial nerve may be abnormal:
- if there is a lesion where several cranial nerves run together either in the brainstem or within the skull (e.g. cerebellopontine angle or cavernous sinus)
- when affected by a generalised disorder (e.g. myasthenia gravis)
- following multiple lesions (e.g. multiple sclerosis, cerebrovascular disease, basal meningitis).

Abnormalities of cranial nerves are very useful in localising a lesion within the central nervous system.

Examination of the eye and the fields allows the examination of a tract running from the eye to the occipital lobe that also crosses the mid line.

The nuclei of the cranial nerves within the brainstem act as markers for the level of the lesion (see Fig. 5.2). Particularly useful are the nuclei of the III, IV, VI, VII and XII nerves. When the tongue and face are affected on the same side as a hemiplegia the lesion

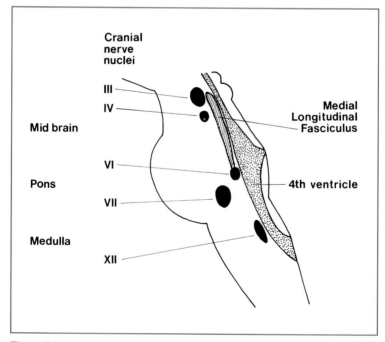

Figure 5.2
Level of cranial nerve nuclei in the brainstem, indicated by Roman numerals.
MLF = Medial longitudinal fasciculus

must be above the VII or XII nucleus respectively. If a cranial nerve is affected on the opposite side to a hemiparesis, then the causative lesion must be at the level of the nucleus of that nerve. This is illustrated in Flow Chart 4.

Multiple cranial nerve abnormalities are also recognised in a number of syndromes:

- unilateral V, VII and VIII — cerebellopontine angle lesion
- unilateral III, IV, V_1 and VI — cavernous sinus lesion
- combined unilateral IX, X and XI — jugular foramen syndrome
- combined bilateral X, XI and XII
  If lower motor neurone = bulbar palsy
  If upper motor neurone = pseudobulbar palsy
- prominent involvement of eye muscles and facial weakness, particularly when variable, suggests a myasthenic syndrome.

The most common cause of intrinsic brainstem lesions in younger patients is multiple sclerosis, and in older patients vascular disease. Rarer causes include gliomas, lymphomas and brainstem encephalitis.

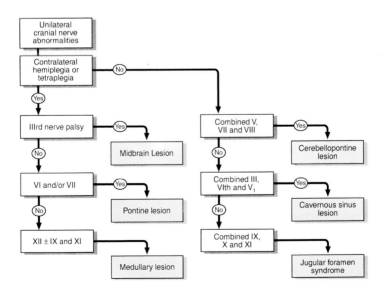

Flow chart 4
Multiple cranial nerve abnormalities

OLFACTORY NERVE

This is rarely tested in clinical practice.

Examination is usually performed to investigate a specific complaint rather than as a screening test. Most recognisable smells require olfaction. Some agents such as ammonia can be recognised by the nasal epithelium and do not require an intact olfactory pathway.

WHAT TO DO

Simple: Take a bedside object, a piece of fruit, an orange, a juice bottle, and ask the patient if it smells normal.

Formal: A selection of substances with identifiable smells in similar bottles are used. Agents often used include peppermint, camphor, rosewater. The subject is asked to identify these smells. An agent such as ammonia is usually included. Each nostril is tested separately.

WHAT YOU FIND

○ The patient is able to identify smells appropriately — *normal*
○ The patient is unable to recognise scents offered but recognises ammonia — *anosmia*. This finding is limited to one nostril — *unilateral anosmia*
○ The patient recognises no smells including ammonia — consider that the loss may not be entirely organic

WHAT IT MEANS

○ **Anosmia in both nostrils**: loss of sense of smell — *common causes*: blocked nasal passages (e.g. common cold), trauma, a relative loss occurs with ageing, Parkinson's disease
○ **Unilateral anosmia** — blocked nostril, unilateral frontal lesion (meningioma or glioma (rare))

THE EYE 1 —
Pupils, Acuity, Fields

BACKGROUND

Examination of the eye can provide very many important diagnostic clues for both general medical and neurological diseases.

Examination can be divided into:

a. general
b. pupils
c. acuity
d. fields
e. fundi (next section).

b. Pupils

The pupillary light reaction
- *afferent*: optic nerve
- *efferent*: parasympathetic component of the third nerve on both sides

Accommodation reaction
- *afferent*: arises in the frontal lobes
- *efferent*: as for light reaction

c. Acuity

Abnormalities may arise from:
- **ocular problems**, such as dense cataracts (lens opacities). Not correctable with glasses but readily identifiable on ophthalmoscopy
- **optical problems**: abnormalities of the focal length of the focusing system in the eye, commonly called long- or short-sightedness. This can be corrected by glasses or by getting the patient to look through a pin-hole
- **retinal** or **retro-orbital abnormality of vision** which cannot be corrected using lenses. Retinal causes are often visible on ophthalmoscopy

It is essential to test acuity with the patient's correct glasses.

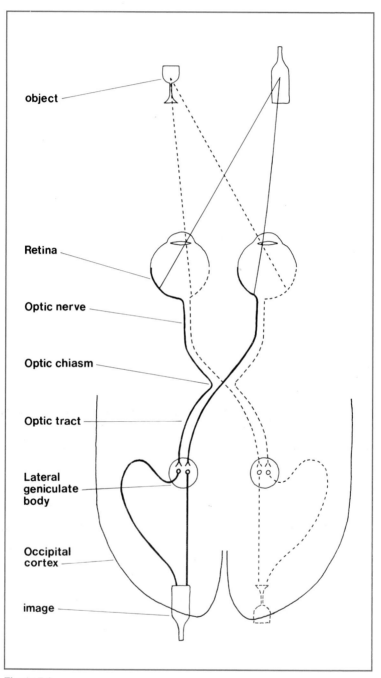

object

Retina

Optic nerve

Optic chiasm

Optic tract

Lateral geniculate body

Occipital cortex

image

Figure 7.1
Visual pathways

d. Fields

The organisation of the visual pathways means different patterns of visual field abnormality arise from lesions at different sites. The normal visual pathways are given in Figure 7.1.

The visual fields are divided vertically through the point of fixation into the temporal and nasal fields. Something on your right as you look ahead is in the temporal field of your right eye and the nasal field of your left eye.

The visual fields are described from the patient's point of view.

Field defects are said to be *homonymous* if the same part of the visual field is affected in both eyes. This can be *congruous* (the field defects in both eyes match exactly) or *incongruous* (the field defects do not match exactly).

Testing the fields is very useful in localisation of a lesion:

Monocular field defects	— lesion anterior to optic chiasm
Bitemporal field defects	— lesion at the optic chiasm
Homonymous field defects	— lesion behind the optic chiasm
Congruous homonymous field defects	— lesion behind lateral geniculate bodies

A. GENERAL

WHAT TO DO

Look at the patient's eyes and note any difference between the two sides

Look at the level of the eyelid; particularly note asymmetry

- an eyelid lower than normal is referred to as *ptosis*; this can be *partial* or *complete* (if eye is closed)
- an eyelid higher than normal, usually above the level of the top of the iris, is described as having *lid retraction*

Look at the position of the eye

Is there protrusion (*exophthalmos*) or does it appear sunken (*enophthalmos*)? If you are considering exophthalmos, it is confirmed if the front of the orbital globe can be seen when looking from above.

Beware the false eye—usually obvious with closer inspection.

WHAT IT MEANS

○ **Ptosis**—*common causes*: congenital, Horner's syndrome (always partial), third nerve palsy (often complete) (see below); *rarer causes*: myasthenia gravis (ptosis often variable), myopathy
○ **Exophthalmos**—*common causes*: most frequently, dysthyroid eye disease—associated with lid retraction; *rarely*: retro-orbital mass
○ **Enophthalmos**: a feature of Horner's syndrome (see below)

B. PUPILS

WHAT TO DO IN A CONSCIOUS PATIENT

(For pupillary changes in an unconscious patient see section 27.)

Look at the pupils
• are they equal in size?
• are they regular in outline?
• are there any holes in the *iris* or foreign bodies (e.g. lens implants) in the *anterior chamber*?

Shine a bright light in one eye
• look at the reaction of that eye—*the direct reflex*—and then repeat and look at the reaction in the other eye—*the consensual reflex*
• ensure that the patient is **looking into the distance** and not at the torch
• repeat for other eye

Place your finger ten centimetres in front of the patient's nose. Ask the patient to **look into the distance and then at your finger**.

Look at the pupils for their reaction to *accommodation*.

WHAT YOU FIND

See Flow Chart 5.

FURTHER TESTING

Swinging light test

What to do
Shine the bright light in one eye and then the other at about one-second intervals. Swing the light repeatedly between the two. Observe the pupillary response as the light is shone into the eye.

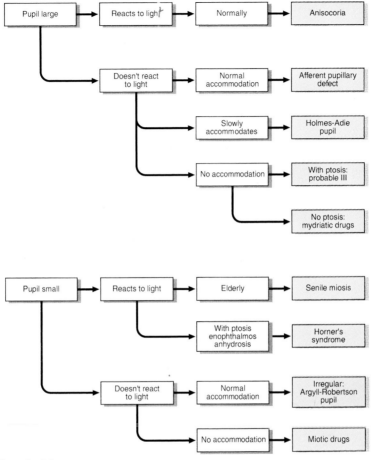

Flow chart 5
Pupillary abnormalities

What you find and what it means
○ The pupil constricts as the light is shone into it repeatedly — *normal*
○ The pupil on one side constricts when the light is shone into it and the pupil on the other side dilates when the light is then shone into it — the side that dilates has a *relative afferent pupillary defect* (often abbreviated to *RAPD*). This is also sometimes called the *Marcus Gunn pupil*
N.B. This lesion is always unilateral

WHAT IT MEANS

○ **Anisocoria**: pupils unequal but normally reacting — *normal variant*

○ **Senile miosis**: normal age-related change

○ **Holmes–Adie pupil**: degeneration of ciliary ganglion of unknown cause; may be associated with loss of tendon reflexes

○ **Afferent pupillary defect**: lesion anterior to the optic chiasm — *common causes*: optic neuritis; *rarer causes*: compression of the optic nerve, retinal degenerations

○ **Relative afferent pupillary defect**: partial lesion anterior to the optic chiasm — causes as for afferent pupillary defects

○ **Horner's syndrome** (meiosis, partial ptosis, enophthalmos and loss of hemifacial sweating): lesion to sympathetic fibres. This may occur:
  – **Centrally**: in the hypothalamus, in the medulla or upper cervical cord (exits at T1) — *common causes*: stroke (N.B. lateral medullary syndrome), demyelination; *rarely*: trauma or syringomyelia
  – **Peripherally**: in the sympathetic chain, the superior cervical ganglion or along the carotid artery — *common causes*: Pancoast's tumour (apical bronchial carcinoma), trauma; *rare causes*: carotid dissection

○ **Argyll–Robertson pupil** — probably an upper midbrain lesion; now very rare — *common causes*: syphilis, diabetes mellitus; *rarely*: multiple sclerosis

C. ACUITY

WHAT TO DO AND WHAT YOU FIND

Can the patient see out of both eyes?

• Ask the patient to **put on glasses** if used
• **Cover one of the patient's eyes**. Test each eye in turn

Acuity can be tested in several ways:

i) using **Snellen's** chart

• Stand patient 6 metres from well-lit chart. Ask him to read down from largest letters to smallest

• Record results: Distance in metres from chart
Distance in metres at which letters should be seen

e.g. 6/6, when the letter is read at the correct distance, or 6/60 when the largest letter (normally seen at 60 m) is read at 6 m

N.5.
Boat, house, horse, cat, cabbage, man, trousers, yellow.

N.6.
Eye, ear, earth, lion, lying, road, green, dog.

N.8.
Bird, wall, silver, tower, train, gorse.

N.10.
Snail, sail, blue, jacket, clam, jockey.

N.12.
Car, crow, grey, bracket, scarlet.

N.14.
White, bank, turbot, jewel.

N.18.
Play, grain, red, goat.

N.24.
Black, frog, tree.

Figure 7.2
Near vision chart

ii) using a **near vision** chart (Fig. 7.2)

- Hold the chart 30 cm from patient and ask him to read sections of print
- Record the smallest print size read (e.g. N6)
- Ensure reading glasses are used if needed

iii) using **bedside material** such as newspapers

- Test as in (ii) and record the type size read (e.g. headlines only, all print)

If unable to read largest letters
See if patient can:
i) **count fingers**. Ask how many fingers you are holding up
ii) **see hand movements**. Ask him to say when you move your hand in front of his eye
iii) **perceive light**. Ask him to say when you shine a light in his eye

Ask the patient to **look through a pin hole** made in a card
- if acuity improves the visual impairment is refractive in origin and not from other optical or neurological causes

WHAT IT MEANS

○ **Reduced acuity correctable by pinhole or glasses**: ocular defect.
○ **Reduced acuity not correctable**: classified according to site in visual pathway

---

Anterior

    Corneal lesion — ulceration, oedema
    Cataract
    Macular degeneration — especially age related
    Retinal haemorrhage or infarct
    Optic neuropathy — inflammatory (MS)
                          — ischaemic
                          — compressive
    Retrochiasmal — macula-splitting field defect (see below)
    Bilateral occipital lesions — cortical blindness

Posterior

D. FIELDS

WHAT TO DO

Assess major field defects

- Ask patient to look with both eyes at your eyes
- Put your hands out on both sides approximately 50 cm apart and approximately 30 cm above eye level. Extend your index finger (Fig. 7.3). Your fingers should now be in the patient's upper temporal fields on both sides.
- Ask the patient to indicate which index finger you move — right, left or both
- Repeat with hands approximately 30 cm below eye level.

If one side is ignored when both fingers are moved together but is seen when moved by itself then there is *visual inattention.*

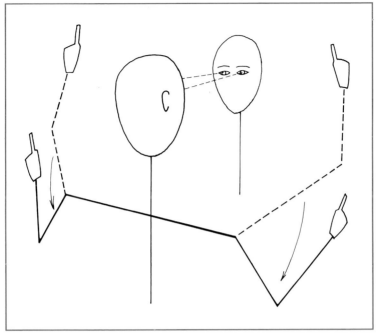

Figure 7.3
Screening for gross visual field defects

Test each eye individually

What to test with?

Large objects are more easily seen than small objects, white objects are more easily seen than red, so fields will vary according to size and colour of target used.

Central vision is colour (cones) and peripheral vision is monochrome (rods).

Use a white hatpin for screening for peripheral visual field defects. Red pins are used to assess defects of central vision and are a more sensitive test for other field defects.

- Sit just under one arm's length away from patient at the same level
- Cover the patient's right eye and ask him to look at your right eye with his left eye. This is so you are certain of his point of fixation throughout the test
- Tilt the patient's head to get the eyebrows and nose out of the way
- Imagine a sphere of radius 30 cm centred on the patient's eye

- **Bring a white pin in towards the line of fixation along an arc** of the sphere (Fig. 7.4)
  - Ensure the pin cannot be seen where you start (usually behind the plane of the eyes). Ask the patient to tell you when he first sees the pin
  - Initially bring the pin **slowly** from four directions, north east, north west, south east and south west (where north/south is the vertical)
  - The field immediately around the fixation point is provided by the macula
- When using a red pin ask the patient to tell you when the pin is seen **as red**. Ensure the pin is midway between your eye and the patient's eye and then compare patient's field to red with your own

Once you find a field defect
Define the edges
Bring the pin from where it cannot be seen to where it can be seen (N.B. the edges are often vertical or horizontal — see Flow Chart 6)

When there is a homonymous hemianopia
The macula needs to be tested

Bring the pin horizontally from the side with the defect towards the point of fixation.
- if the pin is seen before it gets to the midline there is macular sparing
- if the pin is only seen once it crosses the midline there is no macular sparing

Describe the field loss from the patient's point of view.

Central field defects — *scotomas* — and the *blind spot* (the field defect produced by the optic disc) are usually found using a red pin.

Hint: If a patient complains of a hole in his visual field it is often easier to give him the pin and ask him to place it in the hole in his vision.

To find the blind spot move the pin from the point of fixation half way between you, laterally along the horizontal meridian till you find your own blind spot. Ask the patient to tell you when the pin disappears.

Common mistakes
- upper temporal field defects: *eyebrows*
- lower nasal field defects: *nose*
- patient moves eyes ('cheats') *looking to one side: long-standing homonymous hemianopia* on that side

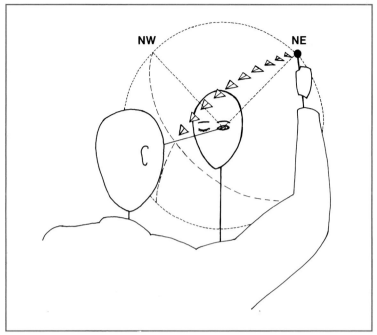

Figure 7.4
Testing peripheral visual fields

WHAT YOU FIND

See Flow Chart 6.

(i) Defect limited to one eye

Constricted field

○ **Tubular vision**—size of constricted field remains the same regardless of distance of the test object from the eye

○ **Scotoma**—a hole in the visual field—described by its site, for example *central* or *centrocecal* (defect connecting the fixation point to the blind spot) and shape (e.g. *round* or *ring-shaped*)

○ **Altitudinal defect**—a lesion confined to either upper or lower half of visual field but crossing the vertical meridian

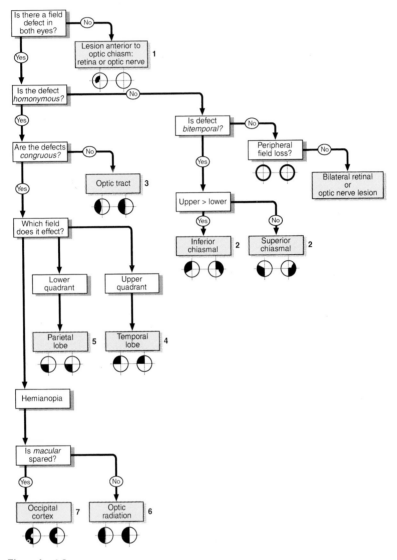

Flow chart 6
Field defects

(ii) Defect affecting both eyes

○ **Bitemporal hemianopias**—defect in the temporal fields of both eyes. Note carefully if upper or lower quadrant more marked
○ **Homonymous quadrantanopias**—defect in the same quadrant of vision of both eyes. Classified as *congruous* or *incongruous* (see above)
○ **Homonymous hemianopias**—defect in the same hemifield in both eyes. Classified as according to degree of functional preservation in affected field (e.g. able to see moving targets) whether *congruous* or *incongruous* and whether *macula-sparing* or not
○ **Others**, including bilateral defects as described in (i)

Before continuing your examination **describe your findings**, e.g. 'This man has normal pupillary response to light and accommodation. His visual acuities are 6/6 on the right and 6/12 on the left. He has a right homonymous hemianopia which is congruous and macula-sparing.'

WHAT IT MEANS

See Flow Chart 6 and Figure 7.5.
(i) *Defect limited to one eye*—indicates ocular, retinal or optic nerve pathology
   ○ **Constricted field**—chronic papilloedema, chronic glaucoma
   ○ **Tubular vision**: does not indicate organic disease—suggests hysteria
   ○ **Scotoma**—multiple sclerosis, toxic optic neuropathy, ischaemic optic neuropathy, retinal haemorrhage or infarct
   ○ **Altitudinal defects**—suggest vascular cause (retinal infarcts or ischaemic optic neuropathy)

(ii) *Defect affecting both eyes*—indicates a lesion at or behind the optic chiasm, or bilateral prechiasmal lesions
   ○ **Bitemporal hemianopias**
      – *Upper quadrant > lower*—inferior chiasmal compression, commonly a pituitary adenoma
      – *Lower quadrant > upper*—superior chiasmal compression, commonly a craniopharyngioma
   The common causes for the lesions referred to below are cerebral infarcts, haemorrhages or tumours.
   ○ **Homonymous quadrantanopias**
      – *Upper*—temporal lobe lesion
      – *Lower*—parietal lobe lesion
   ○ **Homonymous hemianopias**
      – *Incongruous*—lesion of the optic tract
      – *Congruous*—lesion behind the lateral geniculate body
      – *Macula-sparing*—lesion of the occipital cortex (or partial lesion of optic tract or radiation)

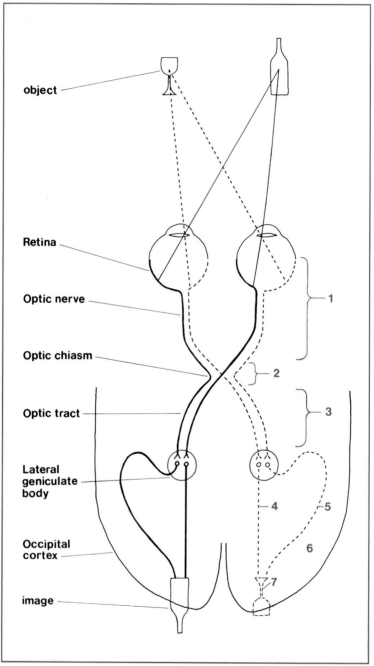

object

Retina

Optic nerve

Optic chiasm

Optic tract

Lateral geniculate body

Occipital cortex

image

Figure 7.5
Visual pathways with sites of lesions marked — numbers match those in flow chart

8

THE EYE 2: Fundi

BACKGROUND

The ophthalmoscope provides a light source and an optical system to allow examination of the fundus (Fig. 8.1).

Moving parts: On/off switch, usually with brightness control

                       Focus ring (occasionally two)

                       Sometimes a beam selector

                       Sometimes a dust cover

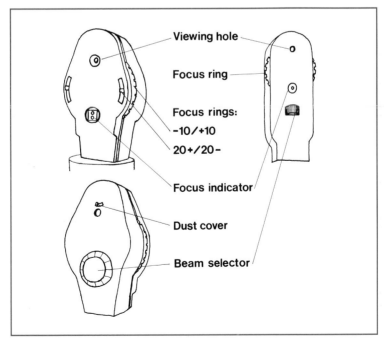

Figure 8.1
The parts of two commonly used ophthalmoscopes

The **focus ring** is used to correct a) for your vision and b) for the patient's vision.

a. If you are short-sighted (*myopic*) and not using glasses or contact lenses you will have to turn the focus dial anticlockwise to focus to look at a normal eye — clockwise if you are long-sighted (*hypermetropic*). Establish what correction you need before approaching the patient.

b. If the patient is myopic turn the ring anticlockwise — if hypermetropic, clockwise.

An oblique view of the patient with his spectacles on tells you if he is long- or short-sighted and gives an idea of severity. If his face is smaller through his glasses he is *myopic*, if his face is larger he is *hypermetropic*. The degree indicates severity.

Beam selector choices a. standard — for general use
b. narrow beam for looking at the macula
c. target (like a rifle sight) to measure the optic cup.
d. green to look for haemorrhages (red appears as much darker)

Common mistakes

- second focus ring, with choices 0, +20 and – 20, is not set to 0
- incorrect beam is chosen — or selection ring is left between two selections
- dust cover not removed
- batteries flat (commonest problem)

WHAT TO DO

- **Turn off lights or draw the curtains**
- **Sit opposite the patient**
- Check the focus is set at zero, the light works and is on the correct beam.
- Ask the patient to **look at a particular point in the distance at his eye level** (e.g. a light switch, a spot on the wall).

To examine the right eye (Fig. 8.2)
- Take the ophthalmoscope in your right hand
- Approach the patient's right side
- **Look at his right eye from about 30 cm away** with the ophthalmoscope in the same horizontal plane as his eye, about 15° from the line of fixation. Aim at the centre of the back of his head. Keep out of the line of sight of the other eye
  - The pupil should appear pink, as in bad flash photographs. This is the *red reflex*
  - Opacities in the eye, notably cataracts and floaters, appear as silhouettes. Cataracts usually have a fine web-like appearance

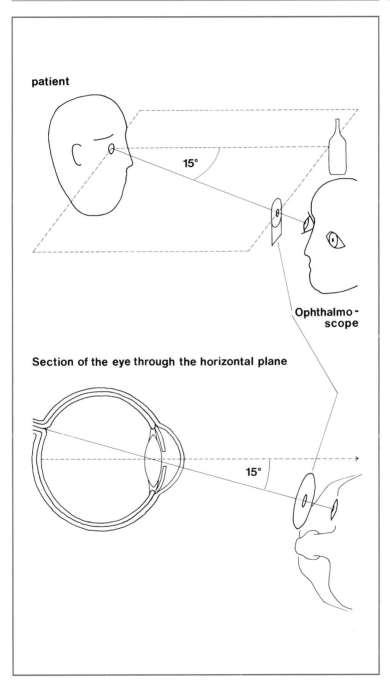

patient

15°

**Ophthalmo-
scope**

Section of the eye through the horizontal plane

15°

Figure 8.2
Approaching the patient with an ophthalmoscope

- **Gradually move in towards the eye**
- Stay in the same horizontal plane aiming at the back of his head. This should bring you in at about 15° to his line of fixation
- Encourage the patient to keep looking at the distant point and not at the light
- Bring the ophthalmoscope to within 1–2 cm of the eye
- Keep the ophthalmoscope at the same level as the patient's eye and the fixation point
- Focus the ophthalmoscope as described above

If the eye is approached as described, the optic disc should be in view. If it is not, focus on a blood vessel and follow it. The acute angles of the branches and convergence of artery and vein indicate the direction to follow. Alternatively, start again.

Hint: it is essential to keep the patient's eye, the point of fixation and the ophthalmoscope in the same plane.

Common problems
- *aphakic eye* (no lens): severely hypermetropic—use high positive lens or examine while patient has glasses on

1. Look at the optic disc

2. Look at the blood vessels

Arteries (light-coloured) should be two-thirds diameter of veins (burgundy-coloured).
- look at the diameter of the arteries
- look at arteriovenous junctions
- look at the pattern of vessels

3. Look at the retinal background

- look adjacent to the blood vessels
- look at all four quadrants systematically

WHAT YOU FIND

1. Optic disc

See Flow Chart 7 and Figure 8.3.

The optic cup is slightly on the nasal side of the centre of the optic disc. Its diameter is normally less than 50% of the disc (see Fig. 8.4).

Optic nerve head swelling can be caused by *papilloedema* or *papillitis*. Papilloedema usually produces more swelling, with humping of the disc margins: not usually associated with visual disturbance (may enlarge blind spot). Papillitis is associated with visual loss, especially central scotomata.

What you find:

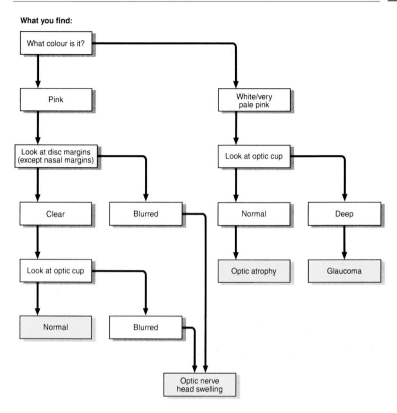

Flow chart 7
Optic disc abnormalities

A swollen optic disc is often difficult to find, with the vessels disappearing without an obvious optic disc.

The difference between papilloedema and papillitis can be remembered:

- you see nothing (can't find the disc) + patient sees everything (normal vision) = *papilloedema*
- you see nothing + patient sees nothing (severe visual loss) = *papillitis*
- you see everything (normal looking disc) + patient sees nothing = *retrobulbar neuritis*

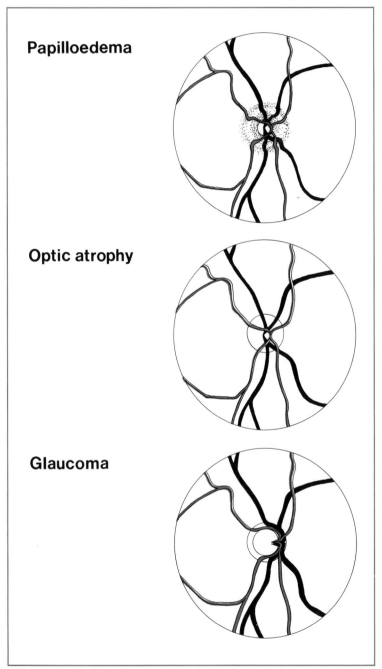

Papilloedema

Optic atrophy

Glaucoma

Figure 8.3
Optic disc abnormalities

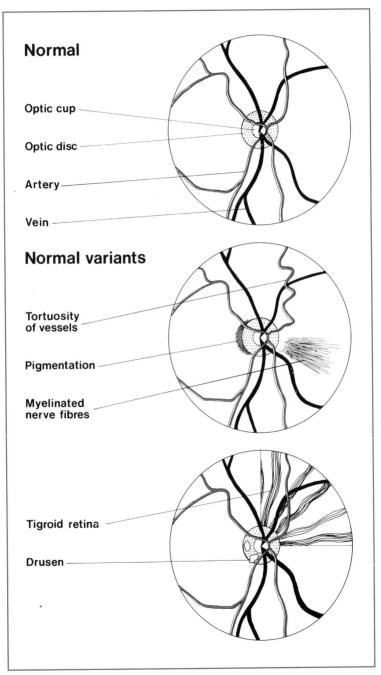

Normal

Optic cup

Optic disc

Artery

Vein

Normal variants

Tortuosity
of vessels

Pigmentation

Myelinated
nerve fibres

Tigroid retina

Drusen

Figure 8.4
Normal variants

Common mistakes and problems

- *blurred nasal margin*: normal, often mistaken for papilloedema
- *temporal pallor*: normally paler than nasal, often misinterpreted as abnormal
- *myopic fundus*: myopic eye is large, so disc appears paler, may be mistaken for optic atrophy
- *hypermetropic fundus*: small eye, fundus appears crowded, mistaken for papilloedema
- *drusen*: colloid bodies that may occur on disc, mistaken for papilloedema
- *pigmentation on disc edge*: normal — may make disc seem pale
- *myelinated nerve fibres*: opaque white fibres usually radiating from disc, may be mistaken for papilloedema

2. Blood vessels

- ❍ **Irregular arterial calibre**
- ❍ **Arteriovenous nipping** — the vein narrows markedly as it is crossed by the artery
- ❍ **Neovascularisation**: new vessels appear as fine frond-like vessels, often near the disc, frequently coming off the plane of the retina — and therefore may be out of focus
- ❍ **Bright yellow object within lumen of artery** — cholesterol embolus

Common mistakes (Fig. 8.4)

- *choroidal artery*: a small vessel running from disc edge towards macula. Mistaken for new vessels
- tortuous vessels: *normal*

3. Retinal background (Fig. 8.5)

General background

- ❍ **Pigmented background**: normal especially in dark-skinned races, if striped called *tigroid*
- ❍ **Pale**: *Clear*:   normal in fair-skinned people, also seen in albinos
        Cloudy: macula appears as 'cherry-red' spot, vessels narrow — seen in retinal artery occlusion

Red lesions

- – **Dot haemorrhages**: microaneurysms seen adjacent to blood vessels
- – **Blot haemorrhages**: bleeds in the deep layer of retina from microaneurysms. Dots and blots are seen in diabetic retinopathy
- – **Flame haemorrhages**: superficial bleed shaped by nerve fibres into a fan with point towards the disc — seen in hypertensive

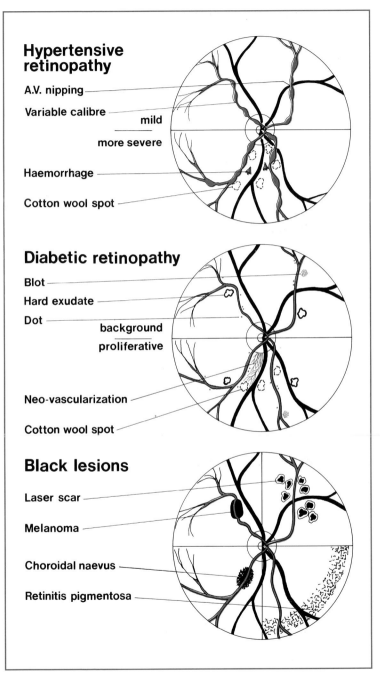

Hypertensive retinopathy

A.V. nipping

Variable calibre

mild

more severe

Haemorrhage

Cotton wool spot

Diabetic retinopathy

Blot

Hard exudate

Dot

background

proliferative

Neo-vascularization

Cotton wool spot

Black lesions

Laser scar

Melanoma

Choroidal naevus

Retinitis pigmentosa

Figure 8.5
Retinal abnormalities

retinopathy; florid haemorrhages seen in retinal venous thrombosis — may be in only one quarter or half retina
- **Subhyaloid haemorrhages**: irregular superficial haemorrhages usually with flat top. Seen in subarachnoid haemorrhages

White/yellow lesions

○ **Hard exudates**: yellowish sharply-edged lesions. May form a ring around the macula — *macular star*. Seen in diabetes and hypertension
○ **Cotton wool spots**: white fluffy spots, sometimes also called soft exudates, caused by retinal infarcts. Seen in diabetes, SLE, AIDS

Black lesions

○ **Moles**: flat, usually rounded lesions — *normal*
○ **Laser burns**: black-edged round lesions, usually in regular pattern. Often mistaken for retinitis pigmentosa
○ **Retinitis pigmentosa**: rare, black lesions like bone spicules in periphery of retina
○ **Melanoma**: raised irregular malignant tumor

WHAT IT MEANS

1. Optic disc

○ **Papilloedema** — *common causes*: raised intracranial pressure (N.B. absence does *not* exclude this); *rarer causes*: malignant hypertension, hypercapnia
○ **Papillitis** — *common causes*: MS, idiopathic
○ **Optic atrophy** – primary—common causes: MS, optic nerve compression, optic nerve ischaemia; *rarely*: nutritional deficiencies, B_{12}, B_1, hereditary
      – secondary—following papilloedema
○ **Deep optic cup**: chronic glaucoma — commonly idiopathic

2. Blood vessels and retinal background

○ **Hypertensive retinopathy (Fig. 8.5)**:
  Stage I: arteriolar narrowing and vessel irregularity
  Stage II: A–V nipping
  Stage III: flame-shaped haemorrhages, hard exudates and cotton wool spots
  Stage IV: papilloedema
○ **Diabetic retinopathy (Fig. 8.5)**:
  Background: microaneurysms, dot and blot haemorrhages, hard exudates
  Proliferative: cotton wool spots and neovascularisation
○ **Cholesterol emboli**: unilateral proximal atherosclerotic lesion — usually internal carotid or common carotid stenosis

9

EYE MOVEMENTS

BACKGROUND

Eye movements are controlled in three ways (Fig. 9.1):

Type of eye movement	Site of control
Command (saccadic)	Frontal lobe
Pursuit	Occipital lobe
Vestibular-positional	Cerebellar vestibular nuclei

In the brainstem the inputs from the frontal and occipital lobes and the cerebellum and vestibular nuclei are integrated so that both eyes move together. Important structures are the centre for lateral gaze in the pons and the medial longitudinal fasciculus (MLF) which runs between the nuclei of the III and IV cranial nerves (in the midbrain) and the VI (in the pons). The III, IV and VI cranial nerves then control the following muscles (Fig. 9.2):

- VI — lateral rectus only
- IV — superior oblique only (SO4)
- III — the others

Abnormalities can arise at any level:

Lesions can be
1. Supranuclear (above the nuclei)
2. Internuclear (connections between nuclei; MLF)   } No double vision (generally)

3. Nuclear
4. Nerve
5. Neuromuscular junction
6. Muscle   } Double vision

Internuclear and supranuclear lesions rarely cause double vision.

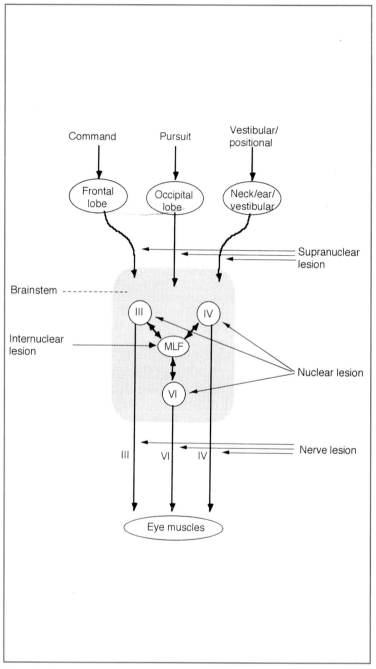

Figure 9.1
Control of eye movements

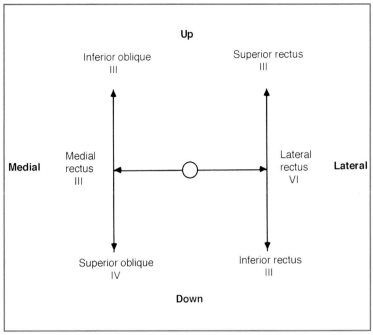

Figure 9.2
Muscles involved in eye movement

Double vision rules
1. Double vision is maximal in the direction of gaze of the affected muscle
2. False image is the outer image
3. False image arises in the affected eye

WHAT TO DO

Look at the position of the head
The head is tilted away from the side of a fourth nerve lesion

Look at the eyes
- note ptosis (see section 6)
- note the resting position of the eyes, the position of *primary gaze*

Look at the position of the eyes in primary gaze
- do they diverge or converge?
- does one appear to be looking up or down—skew deviation?

Perform the cover test (Fig. 9.3)

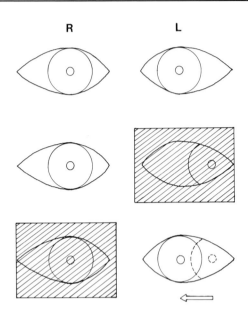

Figure 9.3
The cover test

The cover test: what to do
This is a test for latent squint.

Ask the patient to look with both eyes at your right eye then cover his left eye. Then uncover the left eye rapidly, and cover the right eye. Look to see if the left eye has to correct to look back at your eye. Repeat, covering the left eye and watching the right eye.

The cover test: what you find
If one eye has to correct as it is uncovered this indicates the patient has a *latent strabismus* (squint), which can be classified as divergent or convergent.

The cover test: what it means
○ **Latent squint**: congenital squint usually in the weaker eye (and myopia in childhood) — common

Test the eye movements to pursuit
- Hold a pen vertically about 50 cm away from the patient in the centre of his gaze. Ask him to follow it with his eyes without moving his head and to tell you if he sees double. Hold his chin lightly to prevent head movement
- **Move the pen slowly. Ask the patient to tell you if he sees double**
  - from side to side
  - up and down from the centre
  - up and down at the extreme of lateral gaze
- Ensure the patient's nose does not prevent the pen being seen at the extreme of lateral gaze

Common problems
- the target is too close
- the target is moved too fast
- the patient is allowed to move his head
- in a patient with a hemianopia the target may disappear from the patient's view if moved too fast towards the hemianopia. Thus, in the presence of a hemianopia the target must be moved very slowly

As you do this, watch the movements of the eyes
- do both eyes move through the full range? Estimate the percentage reduction in movement in each direction
- do the eyes move smoothly?
- do both eyes move together?
  If the patient reports he sees double at any stage
  - establish if the images are side-by-side, up and down, or at an angle
  - establish the direction where the images are widest apart
  - in this position briefly cover one eye and ask which image disappears: the inner or outer. Repeat this by covering the other eye (see Flow Chart 8)

Test saccadic eye movements

Ask the patient to look to the right, to the left, then up and down
Observe the eye movements—are they full, do they move smoothly, do they move together?

Look particularly at the speed of adduction.

Test convergence

Ask the patient to look into the distance and then look at your finger placed 50 cm in front of him and gradually bring the eyes in observing the limit of convergence of the eyes.

Double vision

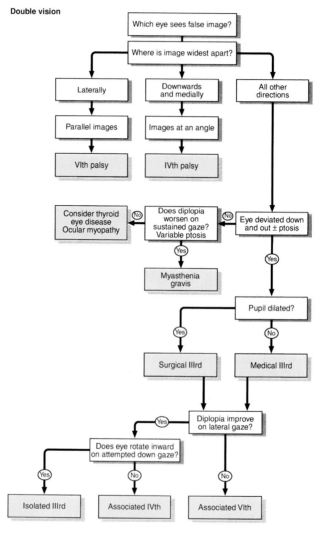

Flow chart 8
Double vision

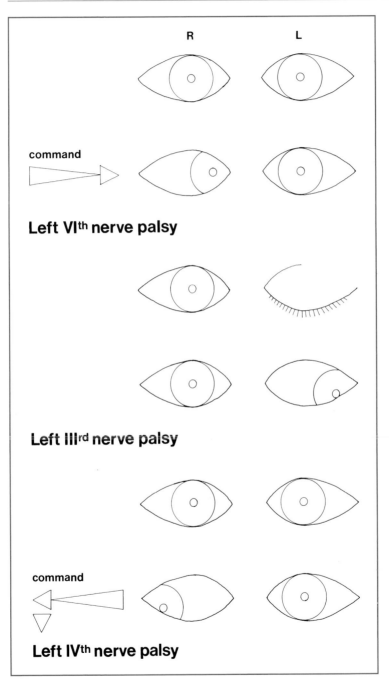

Figure 9.4
Single nerve palsies

Vestibulo-ocular reflex (doll's eye manoeuvre)

This test is performed in patients with a supranuclear or internuclear abnormality.

Ask the patient to look into the distance at a fixed point, then turn the patient's head to the left, then the right and flex the neck and extend the neck.

The eyes should move within the orbits maintaining forward gaze.

WHAT YOU FIND

- ○ **The eyes are misaligned** in primary gaze:
    - The misalignment remains *constant* in all directions for gaze = convergent or divergent concomitant strabismus (squint)
    - *One eye is deviated* downwards and out, with ptosis = third nerve lesion
    - *Eyes aligned in different vertical planes* = skew deviation
- ○ The patient has double vision (see Flow Chart 8):
    Try to answer the following questions:
    Is there a single nerve (VI, III or IV) deficit (Fig. 9.4)?
    - if there is a III nerve deficit, is it medical (pupil-sparing) or surgical (with pupillary dilatation)?
    If not single nerve:
    - is there a combination of single nerves?
    - is it myasthenia or dysthyroid eye disease?
- ○ **Without double vision**
    Compare movements on command, on pursuit and on vestibular positional testing
    - Loss to command only = frontal lesion
    - Loss to pursuit only = occipital lesion
    - Patient does not look towards one side = lateral gaze palsy; check response to vestibulo-ocular reflex testing (Fig. 9.5)
    - Patient does not look up = upgaze palsy
    - Patient does not look down = downgaze palsy
    - Eyes do not move together, with markedly slowed adduction and with nystagmus in the abducting eye = internuclear ophthalmoplegia with ataxic nystagmus (see Fig. 9.6)
    - Eye movement falls short of target and requires a second movement to fixate = hypometric saccades

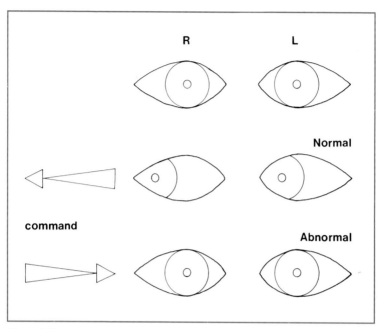

Figure 9.5
Left lateral gaze palsy

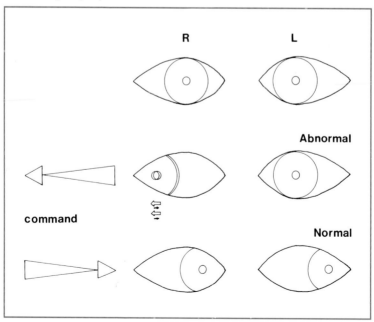

Figure 9.6
Left internuclear ophthalmoplegia

WHAT IT MEANS

○ **Skew deviation**: brainstem lesion — *common causes*: stroke, demyelination — look for associated brainstem signs

○ **Single cranial nerve palsy (III, IV or VI)**: lesion along the course of the nerve or a nuclear lesion — *common causes*:
  - *Medical* — diabetes mellitus, atherosclerosis; *rarely*: vasculitis, Miller–Fisher syndrome (a form of Guillain–Barré syndrome)
  - *Surgical* — (N.B. pupil involvement in III nerve palsy) tumour, aneurysm, trauma, a false localising sign or uncal herniation (III nerve)

  N.B. Posterior communicating aneurysm common cause of a surgical III nerve palsy.

○ **Nuclear lesions**: arise from brainstem pathology including brainstem infarction, multiple sclerosis and, rarely, brainstem haemorrhage and tumour

○ **Lateral gaze palsy**: can arise from:
  - A large frontal or parietal lobe lesion when the patient looks away from the paralysed side (can be overcome by doll's eye manoeuvre)
  - A pontine lesion when the patient cannot look to the non-paralysed side and there may be other pontine abnormalities (facial weakness). Not overcome using doll's eye manoeuvre

○ **Vertical gaze palsy**: lesions in the upper brainstem

  Common causes of lateral and vertical gaze palsies — brainstem infarction, multiple sclerosis, tumour

○ **Internuclear ophthalmoplegia** = a lesion to the medial longitudinal fasciculus — *common cause*: multiple sclerosis; *rarer causes*: vascular disease, pontine glioma

○ **Supranuclear palsy** with preserved positional/vestibular testing: may arise in association with akinetic rigid syndromes (section 24), then referred to as the *Steele–Richardson syndrome* or *progressive supranuclear palsy* and may be seen in other degenerative conditions

○ **Hypometric saccades**: indicates a cerebellar lesion — see section 23

10

NYSTAGMUS

BACKGROUND

Nystagmus is a slow drift in one direction with a fast correction in the opposite direction. It is conventional to describe the nystagmus in the direction of the fast phase.

Nystagmus can be

- *physiological* — oculokinetic nystagmus (as seen in people looking out of the windows of trains)
- *peripheral* — due to abnormalities of the vestibular system in the ear, the eighth nerve nucleus or nerve itself
- *central* — due to abnormalities of the central vestibular connections or cerebellum
- *retinal* — due to the inability to fixate

WHAT TO DO

Ask the patient to follow your finger with both eyes. Move the finger in turn up, down and to each side. Hold the finger briefly in each position at a point where the finger can be easily seen by both eyes.

Watch for nystagmus. Note:

- whether it is symmetrical moving at the same speed in both directions (*pendular nystagmus*) or if there is a fast phase in one direction with a slow phase in the other (*jerk nystagmus*).
- the direction of the fast phase. Is it in the horizontal plane, in the vertical plane or rotatory?
- the position of eye when nystagmus occurs and when it is most marked
- whether it occurs in the primary position of gaze (*second degree*) and if it occurs with the fast phase looking away from the direction of gaze (*third degree*)
- if it affects the abducting eye more than the adducting eye
- if it occurs in one direction only

- if it occurs in the direction of gaze in more than one direction (*multidirectional gaze-evoked nystagmus*)

To decide whether it is central or peripheral note:
- if it persists or fatigues
- whether associated with a feeling of vertigo
- whether it improves with visual fixation

Common mistakes

At the extreme of lateral gaze one or two nystagmoid jerks can be seen normally — ensure target remains within binocular vision.

If found, repeat. If true nystagmus it will appear at less than extreme lateral gaze.

Special test: optokinetic nystagmus (OKN)

This can be tested when a striped drum is spun in front of the eyes and normally evokes nystagmus in the opposite direction to the direction of spin. This is a useful test for patients with hysterical blindness.

Tests for benign positional vertigo are described in section 12.

WHAT YOU FIND

See Flow Chart 9.
Decide whether central or peripheral (see table below)

Central versus peripheral nystagmus

	Sustained	Fatigue	Associated with symptoms of vertigo	Reduced by fixation
Central	+	−	−	−
Peripheral	−	+	+	+

Peripheral nystagmus is not associated with other eye movement abnormalities and usually has a rotatory component.

WHAT IT MEANS

- ○ **Nystagmoid jerks**—*normal*
- ○ **Pendular nystagmus**: inability to fixate—congenital, may occur in miners
- ○ **Rotatory (or rotary) nystagmus**
  - *Pure* rotatory nystagmus = central; peripheral horizontal nystagmus usually has a rotatory component

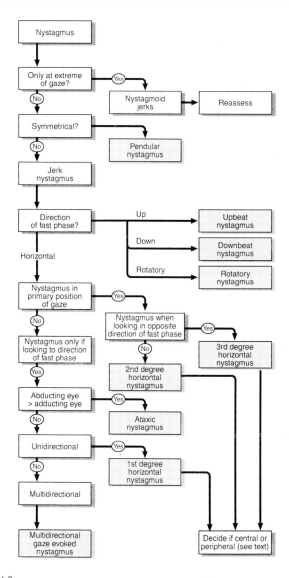

Flow chart 9
Nystagmus

○ **Vertical nystagmus** (rare) — indicates brainstem disease
  – *Upbeat*: indicates upper brainstem — *common causes*: demyelination, stroke, Wernicke's encephalopathy
  – *Downbeat*: indicates medullary-cervical junction lesion — *common causes*: Arnold–Chiari malformation, syringobulbia, demyelination
○ **Horizontal nystagmus** (common)
  – **Ataxic nystagmus** — nystagmus of abducting eye >> adducting eye, associated with internuclear ophthalmoplegia (see section 9) — *common causes*: multiple sclerosis, cerebrovascular disease
  – **Multidirectional gaze-evoked nystagmus**: nystagmus in the direction of gaze, occurring in more than one direction. Always central — cerebellar or vestibular *Cerebellar syndrome* — *common causes*: drugs, alcohol, multiple sclerosis; *rarer causes*: cerebellar degenerations
    Central vestibular syndromes — *common causes*: younger patients — multiple sclerosis; older patients — vascular disease
  – **Unidirectional nystagmus**: second and third degree horizontal nystagmus is usually central; if peripheral it must be acute and associated with severe vertigo. First degree horizontal nystagmus may be central or peripheral:
    peripheral: **peripheral vestibular syndromes** — *common causes*: vestibular neuronitis, Menière's disease, vascular lesions
    central: **unilateral cerebellar syndrome** — *common causes*: as central vestibular syndromes; *rarer causes*: tumour or abscess
      unilateral central vestibular syndrome — *common causes*: as central vestibular syndromes
○ **Unusual and rare eye movement abnormalities:**
  – **Opsoclonus**: rapid oscillations of the eyes in the horizontal rotatory or vertical direction — indicates brainstem disease, site uncertain
  – **Ocular bobbing**: eyes drifting up and down in the vertical plane — associated with pontine lesions

11

THE FACE

BACKGROUND

Facial nerve — VII

Peripheral function can be summarised as:
'Face, ear,
taste, tear'
Face — muscles of facial expression
Ear — tensor tympani and stapedius
Taste — taste anterior 2/3 of tongue
Tear — parasympathetic supply to lacrimal glands
With **lower motor neurone facial weakness** all muscles are affected.
   With **upper motor neurone facial weakness** the forehead is relatively preserved.

Trigeminal nerve — V

- *sensory*: three divisions:
  - ophthalmic (V1)
  - maxillary (V2)
  - mandibular (V3)
  For distribution see Figure 11.1. V1 supplies cornea.
- *motor*: muscles of mastication

WHAT TO DO

Look at the face generally

- is there a general medical syndrome? (e.g. hyper- or hypo-thyroidism, cushingoid, acromegaly, or Paget's disease?)
- is the face motionless?
- are there abnormal movements (see section 24)?

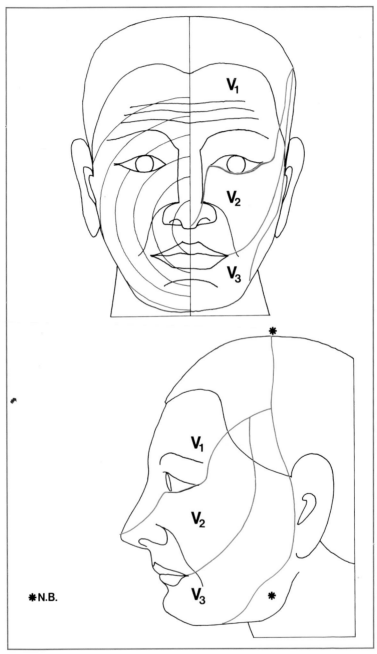

Figure 11.1
Facial sensation: Left side — ophthalmic (V1), maxillary (V2) and mandibular
(V3) divisions of the trigeminal nerve. Right side — muzzle pattern of innervation
— Rings further from the nose go further down the brainstem

FACIAL NERVE: WHAT TO DO

Look at the symmetry of the face
- note nasolabial folds, forehead wrinkles (Fig. 11.2)
- watch spontaneous movements: smiling, blinking

Ask the patient to:
- **show you his teeth** (*demonstrate*)
- **whistle**
- **screw up his eyes** (*demonstrate*)
  Watch eye movement
  Assess the strength by trying to open his eyes with your fingers
- **look up at the ceiling**
Look out for symmetrical movement
Compare strength of forehead and lower face
In LMN lesions you can see the eye turn upwards on attempted closure — *Bell's phenomenon*

Common mistakes
- *mild facial asymmetry without weakness* — normal — ask the patient to look in mirror
- ptosis is *not* due to weakness of muscles supplied by VII

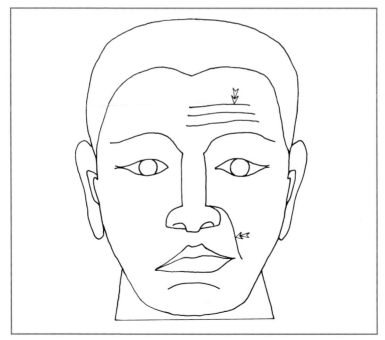

Figure 11.2
Right-sided lower motor neurone VII — note absent facial lines, droopy mouth

Other functions of facial nerves

Look at the external auditory meatus—cutaneous distribution of VII. Note any vesicles suggestive of Herpes zoster.

Provides taste to anterior 2/3 of tongue—taste is rarely tested and requires saline solution and sugar solution. A cotton bud is dipped in the solution and applied to the tongue and the patient is required to identify it. Test each side of the anterior 2/3 and the posterior 1/3.

FACIAL NERVE: WHAT YOU FIND

See Flow Chart 10.

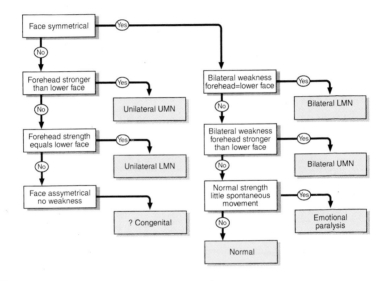

Flow chart 10
Facial nerve abnormalities

FACIAL NERVE: WHAT IT MEANS

○ **Unilateral LMN weakness**: lesion of the facial nerve or its nucleus in the pons—*common cause*—*Bell's palsy*; *more rarely*: pontine vascular accidents, lesions at the cerebellopontine angle, herpetic infections (Ramsey Hunt syndrome—note vesicles in external auditory meatus), lesions in its course through the temporal bone, parotid tumours.

○ **Bilateral LMN weakness** — *common causes*: sarcoidosis, Guillain–Barré syndrome; *rarer causes*: myasthenia gravis can produce bilateral fatiguable facial weakness (neuromuscular junction); myopathies can produce bilateral facial weakness (N.B. dystrophia myotonica and fascio-scapulo-humeral dystrophy)

○ **Unilateral UMN** — cerebrovascular accidents, demyelination, tumours — may be associated with ipsilateral hemiplegia (supratentorial lesions) or contralateral hemiplegia (brainstem lesions)

○ **Bilateral UMN** — pseudobulbar palsy, motor neurone disease

○ **Emotional paralysis** — parkinsonism

TRIGEMINAL NERVE: WHAT TO DO

Motor

Test muscles of mastication (trigeminal nerve — motor)

Look at side of the face:
Is there wasting of the temporalis muscle

Ask the patient to clench his teeth
Feel the masseter and temporalis muscles

Ask the patient to push his mouth open against your hand
Resist his jaw opening with your hand under his chin. Note if the jaw deviates to one side

Jaw jerk — ask the patient to let his mouth hang loosely open. Place your finger on his chin. Percuss your finger with the patella hammer. Feel and observe the jaw movement.

Sensory

Test facial sensation (trigeminal nerve — sensory)
(See section 19 for general comments on sensory testing)

Test light touch and pinprick in each division on both sides: V1: forehead, V2: cheek, V3: lower lip (see Fig. 11.1)

Compare one side to the other. *If abnormal*, test temperature.

If sensory deficit is found determine its edges, moving from abnormal to normal.

THE CORNEAL REFLEX (afferent: ophthalmic branch of V; efferent: VII):

- Ask the patient to look up and away from you. Bring a piece of cotton wool twisted to a point in to touch the cornea from the side
- Watch *both* eyes close
- If there is a unilateral facial palsy the sensation of the cornea can be demonstrated if the opposite eye is watched

Common mistakes:
- the conjunctiva is touched instead of the cornea (Fig. 11.3)

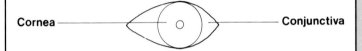

Cornea ——————— Conjunctiva

Figure 11.3
Coreal reflex: Touch the cornea!

- mildly inhibited in contact lens wearers
- cotton wool brought in too quickly acts as a menacing stimulus to provoke a blink

Corneal reflex:

Following corneal stimulation:
- ○ Failure of either side of face to contract = V1 lesion
- ○ Failure of only one side to contract = VII lesion
- ○ Subjective reduction in corneal sensation = partial V1
Absent corneal reflex can be an early and objective sign of sensory trigeminal lesion.

TRIGEMINAL NERVE: WHAT YOU FIND

Motor

○ Wasting of temporalis and masseter: rare — *causes*: myotonic dystrophy, motor neurone disease, facio-scapulo-humeral dystrophy
○ Weakness of — jaw closure — very rare
        — jaw opening: jaw deviates to the side of the lesion — *causes*: unilateral lesion of motor V

Jaw jerk

○ No movement — *absent jaw jerk*
○ Minimal movement — *present normal jaw jerk*
○ Brisk movement — *brisk jaw jerk*

Sensory

○ *Impairment or loss in one or more divisions on one side* (see Fig. 11.1): of light touch or pinprick and temperature or both
○ *Unilateral facial loss*: one or all modalities
○ *Muzzle loss of pinprick and temperature*
○ *Unilateral area of sensory loss* not in distribution of whole division
○ *Trigger zone that produces facial pain*

N.B. 1. Angle of jaw is *not* supplied by the trigeminal but by the greater auricular (C2)

   2. The trigeminal innervates the scalp to the vertex not just to the hair line.

WHAT IT MEANS

○ **Loss of all modalities in one or more divisions**:
   – *Lesion in sensory ganglion* — most commonly Herpes zoster
   – *Lesion of division during intracranial course* — V1 cavernous sinus (associated III, IV, VI) or orbital fissure, V2 trauma, V3 basal tumours (usually associated motor V)
○ **Loss of sensation in all divisions in all modalities**:
   – Lesion of the geniculate ganglion, sensory root or sensory nucleus — lesions of cerebellopontine angle (associated VII, VIII), basal meningitis (e.g. sarcoid, carcinoma)
○ **Loss of light touch only**
   – With ipsilateral hemisensory loss of light touch — contralateral parietal lobe lesion
   – With no other loss — sensory root lesion in pons
○ **Loss of pinprick and temperature** with associated contralateral loss of these modalities on the body — ipsilateral brainstem lesion

○ **Loss of sensation in muzzle distribution**: lesion of descending spinal sensory nucleus with lowest level outermost—syringomyelia, demyelination

○ **Area of sensory loss on cheek or lower jaw**: damage to branches of V2 or V3 infiltration by metastases

○ **Trigger area**: trigeminal neuralgia

12

AUDITORY NERVE

There are two components: auditory and vestibular.

AUDITORY

WHAT TO DO

Test the hearing

Test one ear at a time. Block the opposite ear—either cover with hand or produce a blocking white noise—e.g. crumpling paper.

Hold your watch by his ear. Discover how far away from the ear it is still heard. Alternative sounds are whispering or rubbing your fingers together. Increase in volume to normal speech or loud speech till your patient hears.

If the hearing in one ear is reduced perform Rinne's and Weber's tests.

Rinne's test
- Hold 516 Hz tuning fork on mastoid process (bone conduction (BC)) and then in the front of the ear (air conduction (AC))
- Ask the patient which is louder

Weber's test
- Hold the 516 Hz tuning fork on the vertex of the head
- Ask which ear it is louder in, the good ear or the deaf ear

WHAT YOU FIND

	Rinne test in deaf ear	Weber test
Conductive deafness	BC > AC	deaf ear
Sensorineural deafness	AC > BC	good ear

N.B. With complete sensorineural deafness in one ear, bone conduction from the other ear will be better than air conduction.

WHAT IT MEANS

○ **Conductive deafness** — *common causes*: middle ear disease, external auditory meatus obstruction, e.g. wax
○ **Sensorineural deafness:**
  ○ *Lesion of the cochlea* — otosclerosis, Ménière's disease, drug- or noise-induced damage
  ○ *Lesions in the nerve* — meningitis, cerebellopontine angle tumours, trauma
  ○ *Lesions in the nucleus in the pons* — vascular or demyelinating lesions

VESTIBULAR

Gait

See section 4. Always test heel-toe walking. Gait is unsteady, veering to the side of the lesion.

Nystagmus

See section 10. Vestibular nystagmus is associated with vertigo, horizontal and unidirectional. It may be positional.

Caloric test (normally performed in a test laboratory)

Patient is lying down with head on a pillow at 30° so the lateral semicircular canal is vertical.

Cool water (30°C) is instilled into one ear over 40 seconds (usually about 250 ml). The patient is asked to look straight ahead and the eyes are watched. This is repeated in the other ear, and then in each ear with warm water (44°C).

CALORIC TESTING: WHAT YOU FIND

○ Normal responses: *cold water* — nystagmus fast-phase away from stimulated ear
  warm water — nystagmus fast-phase towards stimulated ear
○ Reduced response to cold and warm stimuli in one ear: *canal paresis*
○ Reduced nystagmus in one direction after warm stimuli from one ear and cold stimuli from the other — directional preponderance

N.B. In the unconscious patient the normal responses are as follows:
- ○ *cold water* — tonic movement of the eyes towards the stimulus
- ○ *warm water* — tonic movement of the eyes away from the stimulus

(The fast phase of nystagmus is produced by the *correction* of this response which is absent in the unconscious patient.)

CALORIC TESTING: WHAT IT MEANS

- ○ **Canal paresis**: Lesion of the semicircular canal (Ménière's disease) or nerve damage (causes as for sensorineural deafness, plus vestibular neuronitis)
- ○ **Directional preponderance**: vestibular nuclear lesions (brainstem) — *common causes*: vascular disease, demyelination

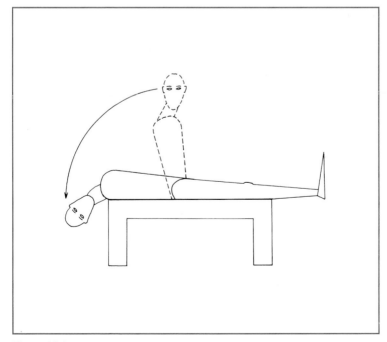

Figure 12.1
Hallpike's manoeuvre

Hallpike's test: used in patients with positional vertigo
- sit the patient on a flat bed so that when he lies down his head will not be supported
- turn the head to one side and ask the patient to look to that side
- the patient then lies back quickly till he is flat with his neck extended with his head supported by the examiner (Fig. 12.1)
- watch for nystagmus in the direction of gaze. Note if this is associated with a delay, whether it fatigues when the test is repeated and if the patient feels vertigo. Repeat for the other side

Hallpike's test: what you find and *what it means*
- ○ **No nystagmus**: normal
- ○ **Fatiguable rotatory nystagmus with delay**: peripheral vestibular syndrome, usually benign positional vertigo
- ○ **Non-fatiguable nystagmus without delay**: central vestibular syndrome

Turning test:
- ask the patient to stand facing you
- ask him to point both arms straight out in front of him towards you
- ask him to walk on the spot and when he is doing this to then close his eyes
- watch his position

Turning test: what you find and *what it means*
He gradually turns to one side, and may turn through 180°. This indicates a lesion on the side he turns towards

13

THE MOUTH

BACKGROUND

Glossopharyngeal (IX):
- *sensory*: posterior 1/3 of tongue, pharynx, middle ear
- *motor*: stylopharyngeus
- *autonomic*: to salivary glands (parotid)

Vagus (X):
- *sensory*: tympanic membrane, external auditory canal, and external ear
- *motor*: muscles of palate, pharynx, larynx (via recurrent laryngeal)
- *autonomic*: afferents from carotid baroreceptors, parasympathetic supply to and from thorax and abdomen

Hypoglossal (XII):
- *sensory*: none
- *motor*: intrinsic muscles of the tongue

MOUTH AND TONGUE: WHAT TO DO

Ask the patient to open his mouth:
Look at the gums
- are they hypertrophied?

Look at the tongue
- is it normal in size?
- are there rippling movements (fasciculations)?
- is it normal in colour and texture?

Common mistakes
- small rippling movements of the tongue are seen if it is protruded or held in a particular position
- fasciculations need to be looked for when the tongue is at rest in the mouth

Ask him to put out his tongue
- does it move straight out or deviate to one side?

To assess weakness:
Ask him to push his tongue into his cheek and test the power by pushing against it: repeat on both sides.

Test repeated movements:
Ask the patient to put his tongue in and out as fast as he can, and move from side to side.

Test speech
See dysarthria — section 2.

MOUTH: WHAT YOU FIND AND WHAT IT MEANS

○ **Gum hypertrophy**: phenytoin therapy
○ **Red, 'beefy' tongue**: vitamin B_{12} deficiency
○ **Large tongue**: amyloidosis, acromegaly, congenital hypothyroidism
○ **Small tongue**: *with fasciculations* = bilateral lower motor neurone lesion; motor neurone disease (progressive bulbar palsy type), basal meningitis, syringobulbia
○ **Small tongue**: *with reduced range of movements* = bilateral upper motor neurone lesion — often associated with labile emotions, increased jaw jerk: pseudobulbar palsy
○ **Tongue deviates to one side** = weakness on the side it moves towards
  – *With unilateral wasting and fasciculation*: unilateral lower motor neurone (rare) — *causes*: syringomyelia, basal meningitis, early motor neurone disease, foramen magnum tumour
  – *With normal bulk*: unilateral upper motor neurone weakness (common) — associated with hemiparesis: strokes, tumours
○ **Tongue moves in and out on protrusion ('trombone' tremor)** — cerebellar disease, essential tremor, extrapyramidal syndromes

PHARYNX: WHAT TO DO

Look at the position of the uvula
• is it central?
If you cannot see the uvula use a tongue depressor.

Ask the patient to say 'Ahh'
Look at the uvula
• does it move up centrally?
• does it move over to one side?

Ask the patient to swallow (provide a glass of water)
• watch for smooth co-ordination of action
• note if there are two phases or any aspiration.

GAG REFLEX: WHAT TO DO

Afferent: glossopharyngeal nerve: *efferent*: vagus
- touch the pharyngeal wall behind the pillars of the fauces (Fig. 13.1)
- watch the uvula: it should lift following the stimulus
- ask the patient to compare the sensation between two sides

PHARYNX AND GAG REFLEX: WHAT YOU FIND

○ Uvula moves to one side: *upper or lower motor lesion of vagus on the other side*
○ Uvula does not move on saying ahh or gag: *bilateral palatal muscle paresis*
○ Uvula moves on saying ahh, but not on gag, with reduced sensation of pharynx: *IX palsy* (rare).

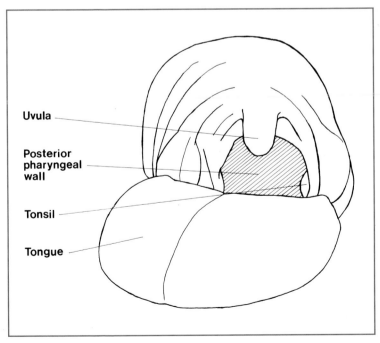

Figure 13.1
The mouth

LARYNX: WHAT TO DO

Ask the patient to cough
Listen to the onset
- explosive or gradual?

Listen to the speech (see section 3)
- are volume and quality normal?
- does the speech fatigue?

Give the patient a glass of water to swallow
Observe the swallowing
- is this smooth or are there two phases with a delay between the aural phase and the pharyngeal phase?
- is it followed by coughing and spluttering?

Laryngoscopy
Direct visualisation of the vocal cords can be obtained by laryngoscopy which allows the position of the vocal cords and their movement to be assessed. This normally requires an ENT opinion.

LARYNX: WHAT YOU FIND

- ◯ Gradual onset cough: Bovine cough—suggests *vocal cord palsy*
- ◯ Bubbly voice and cough—suggests *combined cord palsy and pharyngeal pooling due to tenth nerve lesion*
- ◯ Swallow followed by coughing indicates aspiration due to poor airway protection—suggests *tenth nerve lesion*
- ◯ Unilateral cord palsy—*recurrent laryngeal palsy* or *vagal lesion*

LARYNX: WHAT IT MEANS

- ◯ **Tenth nerve palsy** may be due to lesions in the medulla—look for associated ipsilateral cerebellar signs, loss of pain and temperature in the face on the same side and on the body on the opposite side and an ipsilateral Horner's (lateral medullary syndrome)
  Extramedullary and intracranial look for associated XI cranial, IX cranial nerves
  N.B. Left-sided recurrent laryngeal palsy may arise from mediastinal or intrathoracic pathology.
- ◯ **Bilateral lower motor neurone X** occurs in progressive bulbar palsy (a variant of MND)—look for associated tongue fasciculations and mixed upper and lower motor neurone signs without sensory loss in the limbs

ACCESSORY NERVE

BACKGROUND

The spinal accessory nerve arises from the medulla and has con-
tributions from the spinal route rising from C2 to C4. It is purely
motor and innervates the sternocleidomastoid and the trapezius.

The ipsilateral cerebral hemisphere supplies the *contralateral*
trapezius and the *ipsilateral* sternocleidomastoid. Thus a single
upper motor lesion can give rise to signs on both sides.

WHAT TO DO

Look at the neck
- is sternocleidomastoid wasted or fasciculating?

Look at the shoulders
- are they wasted or fasciculating?

Sternocleidomastoid
Ask the patient to lift his head forward, push head back with your
hand on his forehead. Look at both sternocleidomastoids.

Ask the patient to turn his head to one side, push against his
forehead. Watch the opposite sternocleidomastoid.

Trapezius
Ask the patient to shrug his shoulders, watch for symmetry.
Push down the shoulders.

WHAT YOU FIND AND WHAT IT MEANS

○ Weakness of sternocleidomastoid and trapezius on the same
   side—*peripheral accessory palsy*. Look for associated ipsilateral IX
   and X lesions—suggests a jugular foramen lesion (glomus tumour
   or neurofibroma)

○ Weakness of ipsilateral sternocleidomastoid and contralateral trapezius — *upper motor neurone weakness on ipsilateral side*
○ Unilateral delayed shoulder shrug — suggests *contralateral upper motor neurone lesion*
○ Bilateral wasting and weakness of sternocleidomastoid indicates *myopathy* (such as dystrophia myotonica, fascio-scapulo-humeral dystrophy or polymyositis) or motor neurone disease (look for associated bulbar abnormalities)
○ Unilateral sternocleidomastoid abnormalities: indicate *unilateral trauma, unilateral XI nerve weakness* or *upper motor neurone weakness* (check opposite trapezius)

15

GENERAL

There are five patterns of muscular weakness:
1. **Upper motor neurone (UMN)**—increased tone, increased reflexes, pyramidal pattern of weakness (weak extensors in the arm, weak flexors in the leg)
2. **Lower motor neurone (LMN)**—wasting, fasciculation, decreased tone and absent reflexes
3. **Muscle disease**—wasting, decreased tone, impaired or absent reflexes
4. **Neuromuscular junction**—fatiguable weakness, normal or decreased tone, normal reflexes
5. **Functional weakness**—normal tone, normal reflexes without wasting with erratic power

The level of the nervous system affected can be determined by the distribution and pattern of the weakness and by associated findings (see panel).

Examples of brainstem signs (all contralateral to the upper motor neurone weakness): third, fourth and sixth palsies, seventh lower motor neurone loss, nystagmus and dysarthria.

Hemisphere signs: aphasia, visual field defects, inattention or neglect, higher function deficits.

Mixed UMN and LMN lesions: motor neurone disease (with normal sensation), or combined cervical myelopathy and radiculopathy and lumbar radiculopathy (with sensory abnormalities).

Approach to weakness

Consider **distribution** and whether **upper** or **lower motor neurone** or **muscular**.

Generalised weakness (limbs and cranial nerves)

Diffuse disease of:

Nerve	Polyradiculopathy
Neuromuscular junction	Myasthenia gravis
Muscle	Myopathy

Weakness all four limbs

Upper motor neurone	Cervical cord lesion
	Brainstem lesion
	Bilateral cerebral lesions
Lower motor neurone	Polyradiculopathy
	Peripheral neuropathy
Mixed upper and lower motor neurone	Motor neurone disease
Myopathy	

Unilateral and leg weakness

Upper motor neurone	Hemisection of cervical cord
	N.B. sensory signs
	Brainstem lesion
	N.B. brainstem signs
	Cerebral lesion
	N.B. hemisphere signs

Weakness both legs

Upper motor neurone	Spinal cord lesion
Lower motor neurone	Cauda equina lesion
	N.B. sphincter involvement in both

Single limb

Upper motor neurone	Lesion above highest involved level
	N.B. other signs may help localise
Lower motor neurone	Single nerve = Mononeuropathy
	Single root = Radiculopathy

Patchy weakness

Upper motor neurone	Multiple CNS lesions
Lower motor neurone	Polyradiculopathy
	Multiple single nerves = mononeuritis multiplex

Variable weakness

Non-anatomical distribution	Consider functional weakness

Functional weakness

This should be considered when:
- the weakness is not in a distribution that can be understood on an anatomical basis
- when there are no changes in reflex or tone
- the movements are very variable and power erratic
- there is a difference between the apparent power of moving a limb voluntarily and when power is being tested.

Power when tested is graded conventionally using the Medical Research Council scale (MRC). This is usually amended to divide grade 4 into 4+, 4 and 4–, as below:

5   = normal power
4+ = submaximal movement against resistance
4   = moderate movement against resistance
4– = slight movement against resistance
3   = moves against gravity but not resistance
2   = moves with gravity eliminated
1   = flicker
0   = no movement

Power should be graded according to the maximum power attained, no matter how briefly this is maintained.

WHAT TO DO

Look at the position of the patient overall
Look especially for a hemiplegic positioning, flexion of elbow and wrist with extension of knee and ankle.

Look for wasting
Compare the right side with the left side.

Look for fasciculation: fasciculations are fine subcutaneous movements that represent contractions of a motor unit

Test for tone

Test muscle groups in a systematic way for power

Test reflexes
Develop a system of screening examination (see suggested scheme below). Always
- describe what to do in simple terms
- demonstrate the movements you require
- test simple movements across single joints

- allow the patient to move the joint through the full range before testing power. When testing power look at or feel the muscle contract
- compare the strength of the right side with the left side
- do not be afraid to repeat power tests so as to be certain of your findings

TONE

BACKGROUND

Testing muscle tone is a very important indicator of the presence and site of pathology. It can be surprisingly difficult to evaluate.

WHAT TO DO

Ensure the patient is relaxed, or at least distracted by conversation. Repeat each movement at different speeds.

Arms

Take the hand as if to shake it and hold the forearm. First pronate and supinate the forearm. Then roll the hand round at the wrist (Fig. 16.1)

Hold the forearm and the elbow and move the arm through the full range of flexion and extension at the elbow.

Legs

Tone at the hip

The patient is lying with straight legs. Roll the knee from side to side (Fig. 16.2).

Tone at the knee

Put your hand behind the knee and lift it rapidly. Watch the heel. Hold the knee and ankle. Flex and extend the knee.

Tone at the ankle

Hold the ankle and flex and dorsiflex the foot.

Common problem

Patients fail to relax. This is usually worsened by commands to relax and improved by irrelevant conversations or asking the patient to count down from 100.

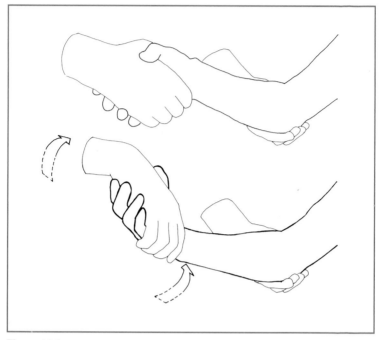

Figure 16.1
Roll the wrist

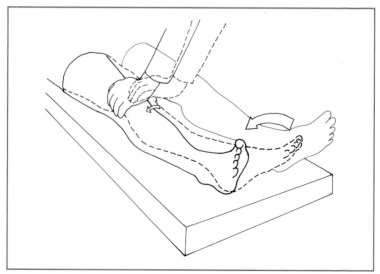

Figure 16.2
Roll the knee

WHAT YOU FIND

O *Normal*: slight resistance through whole range of movements. Heel will lift minimally off the bed
O *Decreased tone*: Loss of resistance through movement. Heel does not lift off bed when knee is lifted quickly
Marked loss of tone = *flaccid*
O *Increased tone*:
  – Resistance increases suddenly ('the catch') heel easily leaves bed when knee is lifted quickly — *spasticity*
  – Increased through whole range, as if bending a lead pipe — *lead pipe rigidity*. Regular intermittent break in tone through whole range — *cogwheel rigidity*
  – Patient apparently opposes your attempts to move his limb — *Gegenhalten* or *paratonia*

Special situations

O **Myotonia** — slow relaxation following action. Demonstrated by asking the patient to make a fist and then release it suddenly. In myotonia the hand will only unfold slowly
O **Dystonia** — patient maintains posture at extreme of movement with contraction of agonist and antagonist. See section 24
O **Percussion myotonia** may be demonstrated when a muscle dimples following percussion with a patella hammer. Most commonly sought in abductor pollicis brevis and the tongue

WHAT IT MEANS

O **Flaccidity** or reduced tone — *common causes*: lower motor neurone or cerebellar lesion; *rare causes*: myopathies, 'spinal shock' (e.g. early after a stroke), chorea
O **Spasticity**: upper motor lesion
O **Rigidity and cogwheel rigidity**: extrapyramidal syndromes — *common causes*: Parkinson's disease, phenothiazines
O **Gegenhalten** or **paratonia**: bilateral frontal lobe damage — *common cause*: cerebrovascular disease
O **Myotonia** (rare) — *causes*: dystrophia myotonica (associated with frontal balding, ptosis, cataracts and cardiac conduction defects) and myotonica congenita. Percussion myotonia may be found in both conditions

ARMS

BACKGROUND

1. Upper motor neurone or pyramidal weakness predominantly affects finger extension, elbow extension and shoulder abduction N.B. elbow flexion and grip are relatively preserved
2. Muscles are usually innervated by more than one nerve root. The exact distribution varies between individuals. Below is a simplified table giving the main root innervations and reflexes. More detailed root distribution is given below.

Nerve roots — simplified root innervations and main reflexes

Root	Movements	Reflex
C5	Shoulder abduction, elbow flexion	Biceps
C6	Elbow flexion (semipronated)	Supinator
C7	Finger extension, elbow extension	Triceps
C8	Finger flexors	Finger
T1	Small muscles of the hand	No reflex

3. Nerves:
   The three nerves of greatest clinical importance in the arm are the radial, ulnar and median nerves.
   The **radial nerve** and its branches supply all extensors in the arm.
   The **ulnar nerve** supplies all intrinsic hand muscles except LOAF.
   The **medial nerve** supplies:
   - L   Lateral two lumbricals
   - O   Opponens pollicis
   - A   Abductor pollicis brevis
   - F   Flexor pollicis brevis
   (N.B. All intrinsic hand muscles are supplied by T1.)

WHAT TO DO

Look at the arms

Note wasting and fasciculations, especially in the shoulder girdle, deltoid and small muscles of the hands (the first dorsal interossei and abductor pollicis brevis).

Test tone (see section 15)

Pronator test

Ask the patient to hold his arms out in front with his palms facing upwards and to close his eyes tightly (*demonstrate*) Watch the position of the arms

What you find and what it means
- One arm pronates and drifts downwards: indicates *weakness on that side*
- Both arms drift downwards: indicates *bilateral weakness*
- Arm rises: suggests *cerebellar disease*
- Fingers continuously move up and down— pseudoathetosis — indicates *deficit of joint position sense*

Basic screening examination

Below a simple screening procedure is outlined. Some further muscle power tests are given afterwards. Perform each test on one side then compare to the other side.

Shoulder abduction
Ask the patient to lift both his elbows out to the side (*demonstrate*). Ask him to push up (Fig. 17.1).

Muscle: deltoid
Nerve: axillary nerve
Root: C5

Elbow flexion
Hold the patient's elbow and wrist. Ask the patient to pull his hand towards his face. N.B. ensure arm is supinated (Fig. 17.2).

Muscle: biceps brachii
Nerve: musculocutaneous nerve
Root: C5, C6
(Trick movement involves pronation of the arm to use brachio-radialis — see below.)

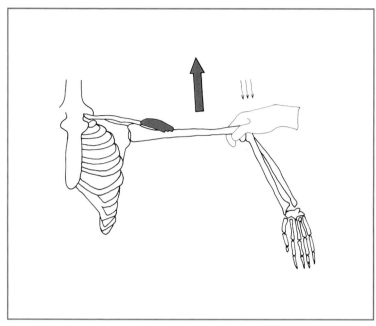

Figure 17.1
Testing shoulder abduction

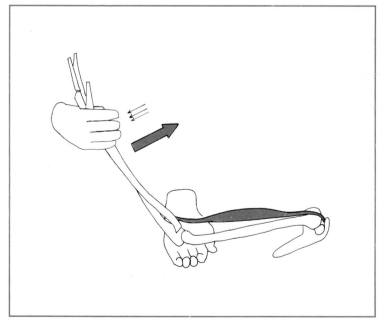

Figure 17.2
Testing elbow flexion

Elbow extension
Hold the patient's elbow and wrist. Ask the patient to extend the elbow (Fig. 17.3).

Muscle: triceps
Nerve: radial nerve
Root: (C6,) C7, (C8).

Finger extension
Fix the patient's hand. Ask patient to keep fingers straight. Press against the extended fingers (Fig. 17.4).

Muscle: extensor digitorum
Nerve: posterior interosseous nerve (a branch of the radial nerve)
Root: C7, (C8)

Finger flexion
Close your fingers on the patient's fingers palm-to-palm so that both sets of fingertips are on the other's metacarpal phalangeal joints. Ask the patient to grip your fingers and then attempt to open the patient's grip (Fig. 17.5).

Muscles: flexor digitorum superficialis and profundus
Nerves: median and ulnar nerves
Root: C8

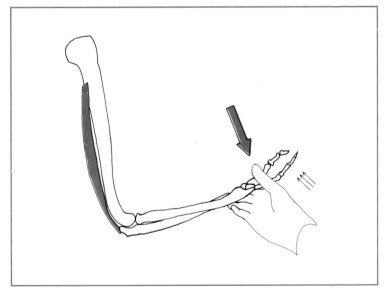

Figure 17.3
Testing elbow extension

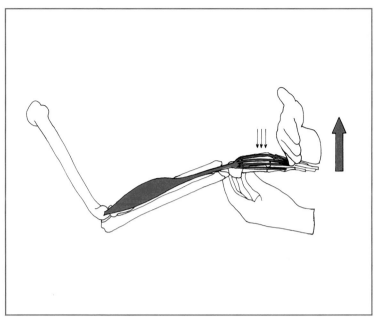

Figure 17.4
Testing finger extension

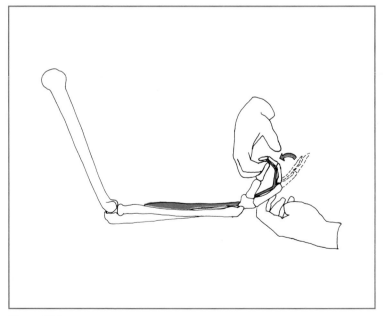

Figure 17.5
Testing finger flexion

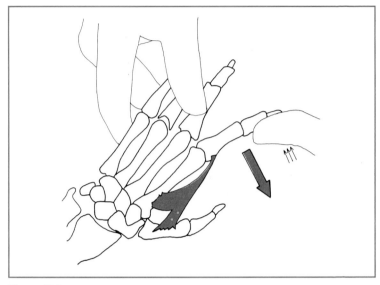

Figure 17.6
Testing finger abduction

Finger abduction

Ask the patient to spread his fingers out (*demonstrate*). Ensure the palm is in line with the fingers. Hold the middle of the little fingers and attempt to overcome the index finger (Fig. 17.6).

Muscle: first dorsal interosseous
Nerve: ulnar nerve
Root: T1

Finger adduction

Ask the patient to bring his fingers together. Make sure the fingers are straight. Fix the middle, ring and little finger. Attempt to abduct the index finger (Fig. 17.7).

Muscle: second palmar interosseous
Nerve: ulnar nerve
Root: T1

Thumb abduction

Ask the patient to place his palm flat with a supinated arm. Ask him then to bring his thumb towards his nose. Fix the palm and pressing at the end of the proximal phalanx joint attempt to overcome the resistance (Fig. 17.8).

Muscle: abductor pollicis brevis
Nerve: median
Root: T1

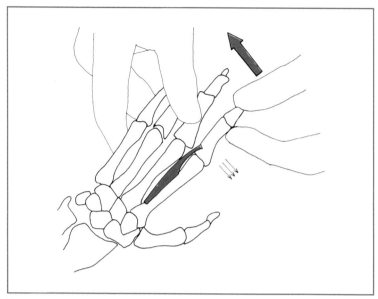

Figure 17.7
Testing finger adduction

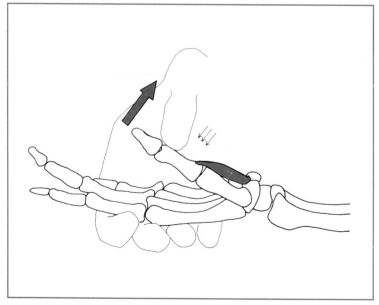

Figure 17.8
Testing thumb abduction

Further tests of arm power

These tests are performed in the light of the clinical abnormality.

Serratus anterior

Stand behind the patient in front of a wall. Ask the patient to push against a wall with arms straight, with hands at shoulder level. Look at the position of the scapula. If the muscle is weak the scapula lifts off the chest wall — 'winging' (Fig. 17.9).

Nerve: long thoracic nerve
Root: C5, C6, C7

Rhomboids

Ask the patient to put his hands on his hips. Hold his elbow and ask him to bring his elbow backwards (Fig. 17.10).

Muscle: rhomboids
Nerve: nerve to rhomboids
Root: C4, C5

Supraspinatus

Stand behind the patient. Ask the patient to lift his arm from the side against resistance (Fig. 17.11).

Nerve: suprascapular nerve
Root: C5

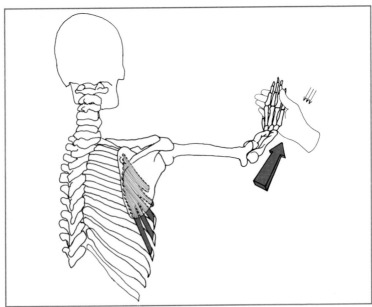

Figure 17.9
Testing strength of serratus anterior

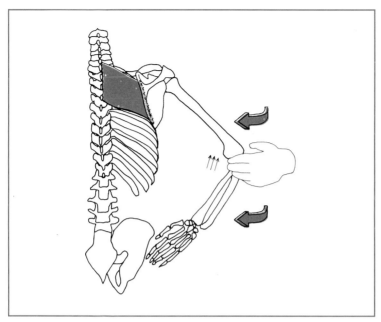

Figure 17.10
Testing strength of rhomboids

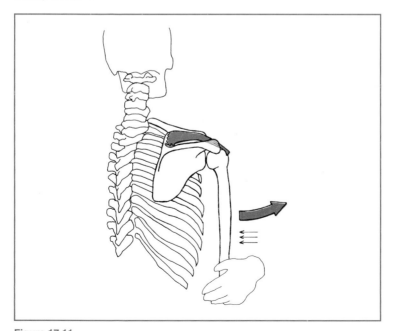

Figure 17.11
Testing strength of supraspinatus

Infraspinatus

Stand behind the patient, hold his elbow against his side with the elbow flexed, asking him to move his hand out to the side. Resist this with your hand at his wrist (Fig. 17.12).

Nerve: suprascapular nerve
Root: C5, C6

Brachioradialis

Hold the patient's forearm and wrist with the forearm semi-pronated (as if shaking hands). Ask the patient to pull his hand towards his face (Fig. 17.13).

Muscle: brachioradialis
Nerve: radial nerve
Root: C6

Long flexors of little and ring finger

Ask the patient to grip your fingers. Attempt to extend the distal interphalangeal joint of the little and ring fingers.

Muscle: flexor digitorum profundus 3 and 4
Nerve: ulnar nerve
Root: C8

WHAT YOU FIND

This will be considered in section 20.

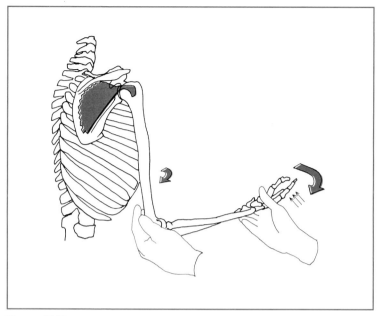

Figure 17.12
Testing strength of infraspinatus

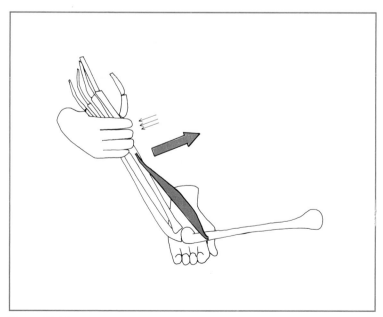

Figure 17.13
Testing strength of brachioradialis

LEGS

BACKGROUND

1. Upper motor neurone or pyramidal weakness predominantly affects hip flexion, knee flexion, foot dorsiflexion
2. Simplified root distribution in the legs

Nerve roots	Movement	Reflex
L1, L2	Hip flexion	No reflex
L3, L4	Knee extension	Knee reflex
L5	Extension of the great toe (extensor digitorum brevis)	No reflex
S1	Hip extension, knee flexion, plantarflexion	Ankle reflex

3. Nerves:
   Femoral nerve supplies knee extension
   Sciatic nerve supplies knee flexion

   Sciatic nerve branches:
   - Posterior tibial branch provides foot plantar flexion inversion and the small muscles of the foot
   - Common peroneal branch supplies dorsiflexion and eversion of the ankle

WHAT TO DO

Look at the legs for wasting and fasciculation
   Note specially the quadriceps, the anterior compartment of the shin, the extensor digitorum and brevis and the peroneal muscles.

Look for the position and for contractures, especially at the ankle; **look at the shape of the foot**, a high arch or pes cavus
   Pes cavus is demonstrated by holding a hard, flat surface against the sole of the foot and a gap can be seen between the foot and the surface.

Power testing screening

Compare the left with the right.

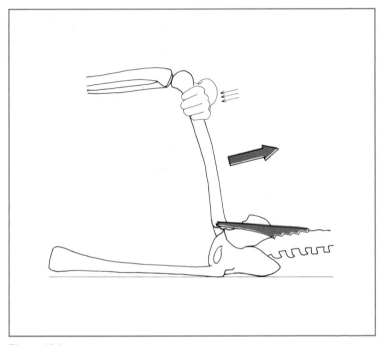

Figure 18.1
Testing hip flexion

Hip flexion

Ask the patient to lift his knee towards his chest. When the knee is at 90° ask the patient to pull it up as hard as he can, put your hand against his knee and try and overcome this (Fig. 18.1).

Muscle: iliopsoas
Nerve: lumbar sacral plexus
Root: L1, L2

Hip extension

The patient is lying flat with his legs straight. Put your hand under his heel and ask him to push down to press your hand (Fig. 18.2).

Muscle: gluteus maximus
Nerve: inferior gluteal nerve
Root: L5, S1

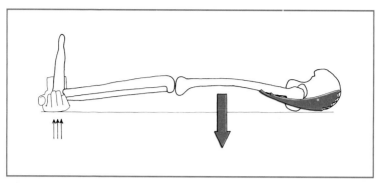

Figure 18.2
Testing hip extension

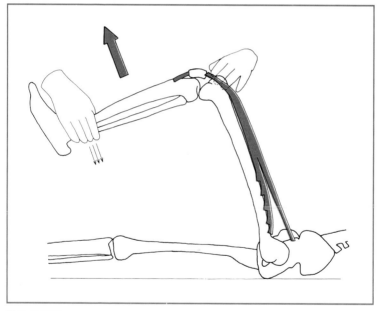

Figure 18.3
Testing knee extension

Knee extension

Ask the patient to bend his knee. When it is flexed at 90° support the knee with one hand and place the other hand at his ankle and ask him to straighten his leg (Fig. 18.3).

Muscle: quadriceps femoris
Nerve: femoral nerve
Root: L3, L4

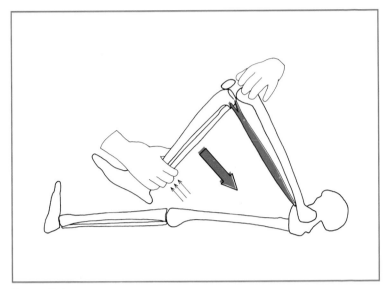

Figure 18.4
Testing knee flexion

Knee flexion

Ask the patient to bend his knee and bring his heel towards his bottom. When the knee is at 90° try to straighten the leg while holding the knee. Watch the hamstring muscles (Fig. 18.4).

Muscles: hamstrings
Nerve: sciatic nerve
Root: L5, S1

Foot dorsiflexion

Ask the patient to cock his ankle back and bring his toes towards his head. When the ankle is past 90° try to overcome this movement. Watch the anterior compartment of leg (Fig. 18.5).

Muscle: tibialis anterior
Nerve: deep peroneal nerve
Root: L4, L5

Plantarflexion of the foot

Ask the patient to point his toes with his leg straight. Try and overcome this (Fig. 18.6).

Muscle: gastrocnemius
Nerve: posterior tibial nerve
Root: S1

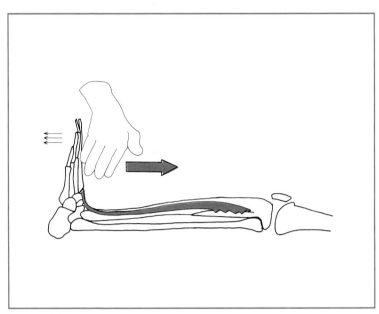

Figure 18.5
Testing dorsiflexion of the foot

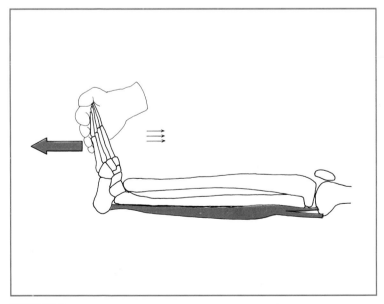

Figure 18.6
Testing plantarflexion of the foot

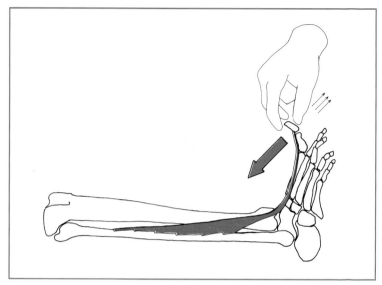

Figure 18.7
Testing big toe extension

Big toe extension
Ask the patient to pull his big toe up towards his face. Try and push the distal phalanx of his big toe down (Fig. 18.7).

Muscle: extensor digitorum longus
Nerve: deep peroneal nerve
Root: L5

Extension of the toes
Ask the patient to bring all his toes towards his head. Press against the proximal part of his toes, watch the muscle (Fig. 18.8).

Muscle: extensor digitorum brevis
Nerve: deep peroneal nerve
Root: L5, S1

Additional tests

Hip abductors
Fix one ankle, ask the patient to push the other leg out at the side and resist this movement by holding the other ankle (Fig. 18.9).

Muscle: gluteus medius and minimus
Nerve: superior gluteal nerve
Root: L4, L5

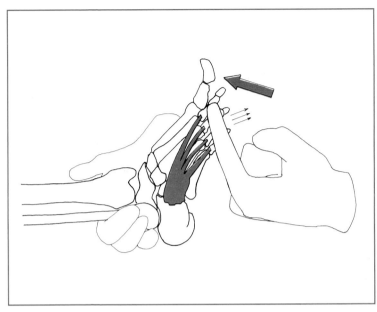

Figure 18.8
Testing extension of the toes

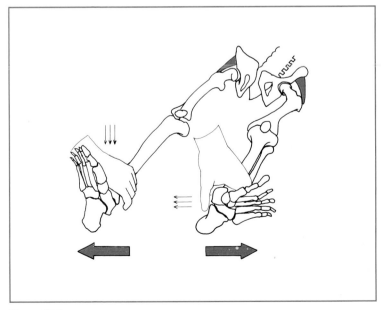

Figure 18.9
Testing strength of hip abductors

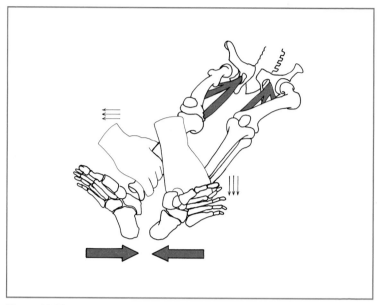

Figure 18.10
Testing strength of right hip adductors

Hip adductors
Ask the patient to keep his ankles together. Fix one ankle and try and pull the other ankle out (Fig. 18.10).

Muscle: adductors
Nerve: obturator nerve
Root: L2, L3

Foot inversion
With the ankle at 90° ask the patient to turn his foot inwards. This frequently requires demonstration (Fig. 18.11).

Muscle: tibialis posterior
Nerve: tibial nerve
Root: L4, L5

Foot eversion
Ask the patient to turn his foot out to the side. Try and then bring the foot to the midline (Fig. 18.12).

Muscle: peroneus longus and brevis
Nerve: superficial peroneal nerve
Root: L5, S1

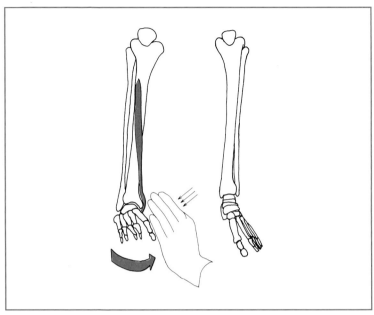

Figure 18.11
Testing inversion of the foot

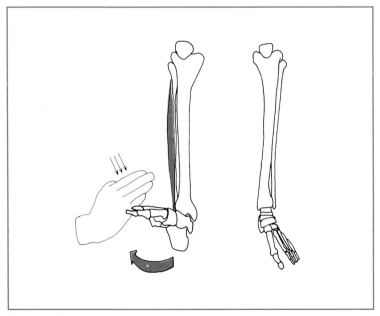

Figure 18.12
Testing eversion of the foot

REFLEXES

TENDON REFLEXES

BACKGROUND

A tendon reflex results from the stimulation of a stretch-sensitive gamma afferent which, via a single synapse, stimulates a motor nerve leading to a muscle contraction. Tendon reflexes are increased in upper motor neurone lesions and decreased in lower motor neurone lesions and muscle abnormalities.

The root values for the reflexes can be recalled by counting (Fig. 19.1) from the ankle upwards.

Reflexes can be graded as follows:

3+   = clonus
2+   = increased
1+   = normal
+/− = obtainable with reinforcement
0   = absent

WHAT TO DO

Use the whole length of the patella hammer, let the hammer swing. Ensure the patient is relaxed. Avoid telling the patient to relax as this is guaranteed to produce tension.

Biceps

Place the patient's hands on his abdomen. Place your index finger on the biceps tendon, swing the hammer on to your finger while watching the biceps muscle (Fig. 19.2).

Nerve: musculocutaneous nerve
Root: C5, (C6)

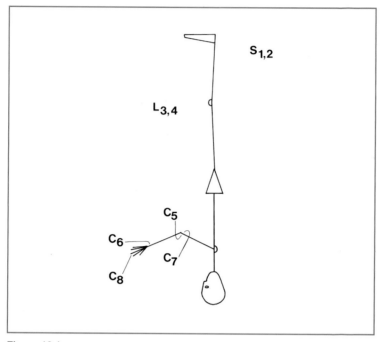

Figure 19.1
Reflex man

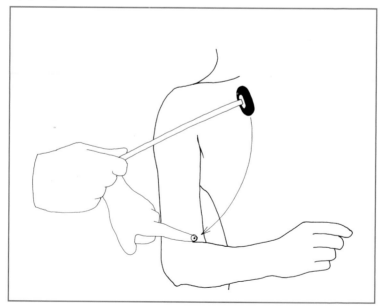

Figure 19.2
Testing the biceps reflex

Supinator

(N.B. Bad name for this reflex, muscle involved is brachioradialis.)

Place the arm flexed on to the abdomen, place the finger on the radial tuberosity, hit the finger with the hammer, watch brachioradialis (Fig. 19.3).

Nerve: radial nerve
Root: C6, (C5)

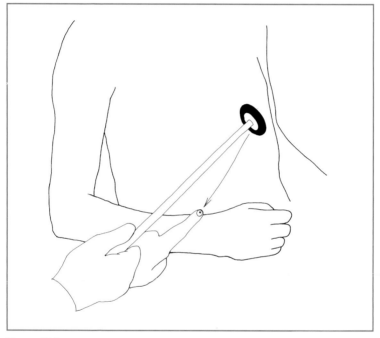

Figure 19.3
Testing the supinator reflex

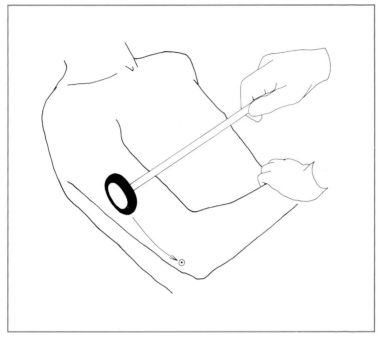

Figure 19.4
Testing the triceps reflex

Triceps
Draw the arm across the chest, holding the wrist with the elbow at
90°. Strike the triceps tendon directly with the patella hammer,
watch the muscle (Fig. 19.4).

Nerve: radial nerve
Root: C7

Finger reflex
Hold the hand in the neutral position, place your hand opposite the
fingers, strike the back of your fingers.

Muscle: flexor digitorum profundus and superficialis
Nerve: median and ulnar
Root: C8

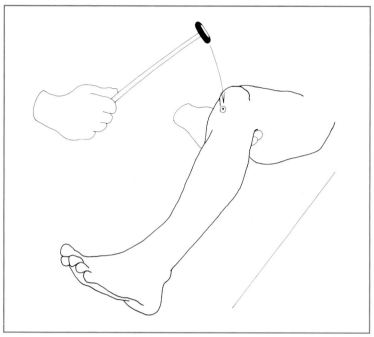

Figure 19.5
Testing the knee reflex

Knee reflex

Place the arm under the knee so that the knee is at 90°. Strike the knee below the patella; watch the quadriceps (Fig. 19.5).

Nerve: femoral nerve
Root: L3–L4

Ankle reflex

Hold foot at 90° with a medial malleolus facing the ceiling. The knee should be flexed and lying to the side. Strike the achilles tendon directly. Watch the muscles of the calf (Fig. 19.6a).

Nerve: tibial nerve
Root: S1–S2

Ankle reflex alternative: With legs straight place your hand on the ball of the foot with the ankles at 90°. Strike with your hand, watch the muscles of the calf (Fig. 19.6b).

Ankle reflex alternative: Ask the patient to kneel on a chair so that his ankles are hanging loose over the edge. Strike the achilles tendon directly (Fig. 19.6c).

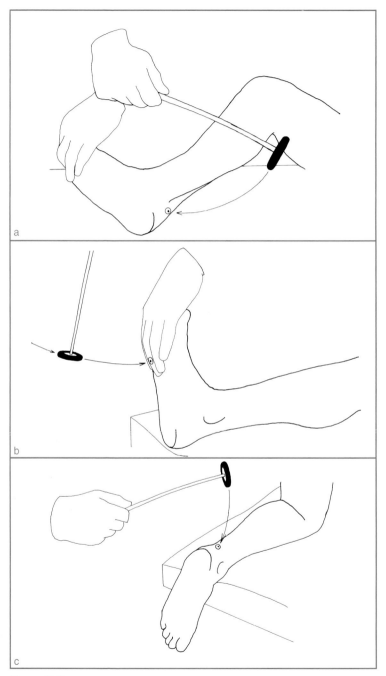

Figure 19.6
The ankle reflex — three ways to get it

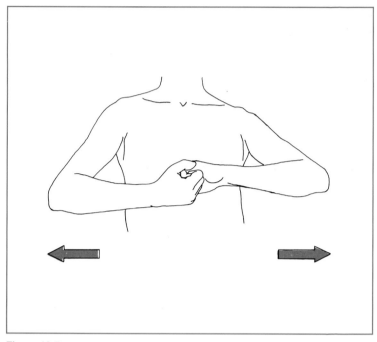

Figure 19.7
Reinforcement

Reinforcement

If any reflex is unobtainable directly ask the patient to perform a reinforcement manoeuvre. In the arms ask the patient to clench his teeth as you swing the hammer. In the legs ask the patient either to make a fist, or to link hands across his chest and pull one against the other, as you swing the hammer (Fig. 19.7).

Common problems

- patient will not relax — ask the patient diverting questions: where the patient comes from, how long he has lived there, and so on
- tendon hammer not swung but stabbed — hold the hammer correctly

Hint: An absent reflex sounds dull — it's worth listening as well as watching.

Further manoeuvres

Demonstration of clonus

At the ankle: Dorsiflex the ankle briskly, maintain the foot in that position, a rhythmic contraction may be found. More than three beats is abnormal.

At the knee: With the leg straight take the patella and bring it briskly downwards; a rhythmic contraction may be noted. Always abnormal.

WHAT YOU FIND AND WHAT IT MEANS

○ **Increased reflex or clonus** — this indicates upper motor neurone lesion above the root at that level
○ **Absent reflexes**:
  – *generalised* — indicates peripheral neuropathy
  – *isolated* — indicates either a peripheral nerve or, more commonly, a root lesion
○ *Reduced reflexes* (more difficult to judge) — occurs in a peripheral neuropathy, muscle disease and cerebellar syndrome
  N.B. Reflexes can be absent in the early stages of severe upper motor neurone lesion — 'spinal shock'
○ **An inverted reflex** — the reflex tested is absent but there is spread to a lower level. The level of the absent reflex indicates the level of the lesion. For example, a biceps reflex is absent but produces a triceps response. This indicates a lower motor neurone lesion at the level of the absent reflex (in this case C5) with upper motor neurone lesion below indicating spinal cord involvement at the level of the absent reflex
○ **Pendular reflex** — this is usually best seen in the knee jerk where the reflex continues to swing for several beats. This is associated with cerebellar disease
○ **Slow relaxing reflex** — this is especially seen at the ankle reflex and may be difficult to note. It is associated with hypothyroidism

ABDOMINAL REFLEXES

WHAT TO DO

Using an orange stick lightly scratch the abdominal wall as indicated in Figure 19.8. Watch the abdominal wall: this should contract on the same side.

Afferents: segmental sensory nerves
Efferents: segmental motor nerves
Roots: above the umbilicus T8–T9, below the umbilicus T10–T11

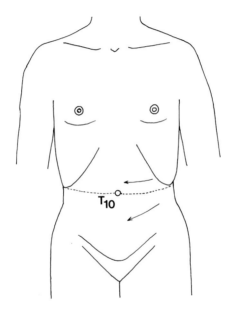

Figure 19.8
Abdominal reflexes

WHAT YOU FIND AND WHAT IT MEANS

○ **Abdominal reflex absent**—obesity, previous abdominal operations or frequent pregnancy, age, a pyramidal tract involvement above that level or a peripheral nerve abnormality

PLANTAR RESPONSE (BABINSKI'S SIGN)

WHAT TO DO

Explain to the patient that you are going to stroke the bottom part of his foot. Gently draw an orange stick up a lateral border of the foot and across the foot pad. Watch the big toe and the remainder of the foot (Fig. 19.9).

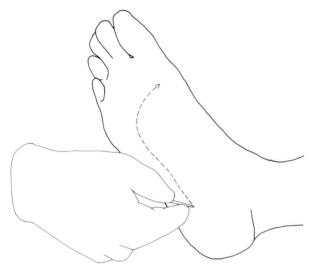

Figure 19.9
Testing the plantar response

WHAT YOU FIND

- ○ The toes all flex—flexor plantar response—*negative Babinski's sign*—*normal*
- ○ Hallux extends, the other toes spread—extensor plantar response or *positive Babinski's sign*.
- ○ Hallux extends, the other toes extend and ankle flexes—*withdrawal response*, repeat more gently or try alternative stimuli (see below)
- ○ No movement—indicates *no response*

(Continued overleaf)

WHAT IT MEANS

○ **Babinski's sign positive** — indicates upper motor neurone lesion

○ **Babinski's sign negative** — *normal*

○ **No response** — may occur with profound upper motor neurone weakness (toe unable to extend); may occur if there is a sensory abnormality interfering with the afferent part of the reflex

Common mistake

Do not place too much weight on the plantar response in isolation. A negative Babinski sign may be found in an upper motor neurone lesion. A positive Babinski which surprises you (one that doesn't fit the rest of the clinical picture) needs to be interpreted with caution — could it be a withdrawal response?

Alternative stimuli (all trying to elicit the same responses)

- stimulus on lateral aspect of foot — *Chaddock's reflex*
- thumb and index finger run down the medial aspect of the tibia — *Oppenheim's reflex*

WHAT YOU FIND AND WHAT IT MEANS

WHAT YOU FIND

Remember:

- ○ **Upper motor neurone pattern**—increased tone, brisk reflexes, pyramidal pattern of weakness, extensor plantar responses
- ○ **Lower motor neurone pattern**—wasting, fasciculation, decreased tone, decreased or absent reflexes, flexor plantars
- ○ **Muscle disease**—wasting (usually proximal), decreased tone, decreased or absent reflexes
- ○ **Neuromuscular junction**—fatiguable weakness, normal or decreased tone, normal reflexes
- ○ **Functional weakness**—no wasting, normal tone, normal reflexes, erratic power, non-anatomical distribution of loss

See Flow Chart 11.

1. Weakness in all four limbs

a. With increased reflexes and extensor plantar responses

- ○ Anatomical localisation—cervical cord lesion or bilateral pyramidal lesions. N.B. sensory testing and cranial nerve signs may be used to discriminate

b. With absent reflexes

- ○ Polyradiculopathy or peripheral neuropathy or a myopathy. Sensory testing should be normal in a myopathy
  N.B. In the state of 'spinal shock' (acute/severe upper motor neurone lesion) reflexes may be absent in an upper motor neurone picture

c. Mixed upper motor neurone (in the legs) and lower motor neurone weakness (in the arms)

- ○ Suggests motor neurone disease (which has *no* sensory loss) or mixed cervical myelopathy and radiculopathy (with sensory loss)

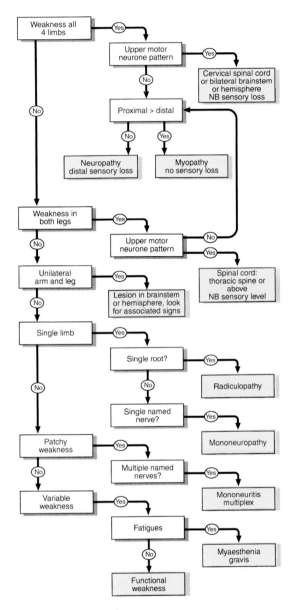

Flow chart 11
Simplified approach to weakness

d. Normal reflexes
○ Fatiguable weakness, particularly with associated cranial nerve abnormalities (eye movements, ptosis, facial muscles)—*myasthenia gravis*
○ Variable weakness, normal tone—consider *hysterical weakness*, if mental state appropriate

2. Weakness in both legs

a. With increased reflexes and extensor plantar responses
○ Suggests a lesion in the spinal cord. The lesion must be above the root level of the highest motor abnormality. A level may be ascertained with sensory signs

b. With absent reflexes in the legs
○ Polyradiculopathy, cauda equina lesions or peripheral neuropathy

3. Unilateral arm and leg weakness

Upper motor neurone lesion in the high cervical cord, brainstem or above
○ contralateral sensory findings (pain and temperature loss) indicate lesion of half ipsilateral cervical cord lesion (Brown–Séquard) (see section 21)
○ contralateral cranial nerve lesions or brain stem signs indicate the level of brainstem affected
○ ipsilateral facial or tongue weakness indicate lesion above brainstem
N.B. Associated cranial nerve, visual field defect or higher function defect may allow more accurate localisation

4. Syndromes limited to a single limb

If upper motor neurone indicates lesion above that level, in spinal cord, brainstem or hemisphere but does not identify level.
  If lower motor neurone, common syndromes seen:

a. Upper limb

Hand
  (i) *Median nerve*—weakness and wasting of thenar eminence abductor pollicis brevis
    Sensory loss—thumb, index and middle finger (section 21)

  (ii) *Ulnar nerve*—weakness with or without wasting of all muscles in hand excepting the LOAF
    Sensory loss—little and half ring finger (section 21)

(iii) *T1 root* — wasting of all small muscles of the hand
N.B. *sensory changes* confined to the medial forearm.

(iv) *Radial nerve* — weakness of finger extension, wrist extension and probably triceps and brachioradialis. *Minimal sensory changes* at anatomical snuffbox. *Reflex loss* — supinator; triceps may also be lost if lesion above spiral groove

(v) Bilateral wasting of small muscles
   – *With distal sensory loss* — peripheral neuropathy
   – *Without sensory loss* — motor neurone disease

Arm

(i) *C5 root* — weakness of shoulder abduction and external rotation and elbow flexion; loss of biceps reflex; *sensory loss* — outer aspect of upper arm (section 21)

(ii) *C6 root* — weakness of elbow flexion, pronation; loss of supinator reflex; *sensory loss* — lateral aspect of forearm and thumb (section 21)

(iii) *C7 root* — weakness of elbow and wrist extension; loss of triceps reflex; *sensory loss* — middle finger (section 21)
N.B. cf radial nerve

(iv) *C8 root* — weakness of finger flexion; loss of finger reflex; *sensory loss* — medial aspect of forearm (section 21)

(v) Axillary nerve — weakness of shoulder abduction (deltoid); *sensory loss* — small patch on lateral part of shoulder (section 21)

b. Lower limb

(i) *Common peroneal palsy* — weakness of foot dorsiflexion and eversion with preserved inversion; *sensory loss* — lateral shin and dorsum of foot (section 21)
N.B. cf L5 root

(ii) *L4 root* — weakness of knee extension and foot dorsiflexion; *reflex loss* — knee reflex; *sensory loss* — medial shin (section 21)

(iii) *L5 root* — weakness of foot dorsiflexion, inversion and eversion, extension of the big toe and hip abduction; *sensory loss* lateral shin and dorsum of foot (section 21)

(iv) *S1 root* — weakness of plantar flexion, and foot eversion; *reflex loss* — ankle reflex; *sensory loss* — lateral border of foot, sole of foot (section 21)

5. Variable weakness

a. Progressively gets worse — consider myasthenia gravis
b. Fluctuates at times giving full power — consider functional weakness

WHAT IT MEANS

Myopathy (rare)

Causes

- **Inherited**—muscular dystrophies (Duchenne's, Becker's, facio-scapular-humeral, myotonic dystrophy)
- **Inflammatory**—polymyositis, dermatomyositis, polymyalgia rheumatica
- **Endocrine**—steroid induced, hyperthyroid, hypothyroid
- **Metabolic**—(very rare) glycogen storage disease (e.g. Pompe's disease), McArdle's disease
- **Toxic**—alcohol, chloroquine, clofibrate

Myasthenic syndromes (rare)

Causes

- **Myasthenia gravis**—usually idiopathic—occasionally drug-induced (penicillamine, hydralazine)
- **Lambert–Eaton syndrome**—paraneoplastic syndrome (usually oat cell carcinoma)

Mononeuropathies (very common)

Common causes

- **Compression** (Saturday night palsy—compressing radial nerve in spiral groove by leaning arm over chair—also reported to affect sciatic nerve after falling asleep sitting on toilet!)
- **Entrapment**, e.g. median nerve in carpel tunnel, common peroneal nerve behind head of the fibula at the knee; more common in diabetes mellitus, rheumatoid arthritis, hypothyroidism and acromegaly
- May be presentation of more diffuse neuropathy

Radiculopathies (common)

Common causes
- **Cervical or lumbar disc protrusion**
  N.B. The root compressed is from the lower of the levels—e.g. an L5/S1 disc compresses the S1 root
  N.B. A radiculopathy may occur at the level of a compressive spinal lesion

Rare causes—secondary tumours, neurofibromas

Peripheral neuropathies (common)

- *Acute predominantly motor neuropathies*: Guillain–Barré syndrome; *very rarely*: diphtheria, porphyria

○ *Subacute sensorimotor neuropathies*: vitamin deficiencies (B_1, B_{12}); heavy metal toxicity (lead, arsenic, thallium); drugs (vincristine, isoniazid); uraemia
○ *Chronic sensorimotor neuropathies*:
  – Acquired: diabetes mellitus; hypothyroidism; paraproteinaemias; amyloidosis
  – Inherited: hereditary motor and sensory neuropathy (Charcot–Marie–Tooth disease)

Mononeuritis multiplex (rare)

○ *Inflammatory*: polyarteritis nodosa, rheumatoid arthritis, systemic lupus erythematosus, sarcoidosis
N.B. may be presentation of more diffuse process

Polyradiculopathy (rare)

Indicates lesion to the many roots. It is a distinct from other peripheral neuropathies because it produces a more proximal weakness. The term is commonly applied to Guillain–Barré syndrome.

Spinal cord syndromes (common)

Sensory findings are needed to interpret the significance of motor signs indicating a spinal cord syndrome—see section 21.

Brainstem lesions (common)

○ **Young patients**—*common causes*: multiple sclerosis
○ **Older patients**—*common causes*: brainstem infarction following emboli or thrombosis; haemorrhage
○ *Rarer causes*—tumours, trauma

Hemisphere lesions (common)

○ **Older patients**—*common causes*: infarction following emboli or thrombosis; haemorrhage; *rarer causes*—tumours, trauma, multiple sclerosis

Functional weakness

Difficult to assess. May be an elaboration of an underlying organic weakness. May indicate hysterical illness. cf functional sensory loss.

GENERAL

BACKGROUND

There are five basic modalities of sensation.

Modality	Tract	Fibre size
Vibration sense Joint position sense Light touch	Posterior column	Large fibre
Pin prick Temperature	Spinothalamic tract	Small fibre

The posterior column remains ipsilateral up to the medulla where it crosses over. The spinothalamic tract mostly crosses within one to two segments of entry (Fig. 21.1).

Vibration sense, joint position sense, temperature are often lost without prominent symptoms.

Light touch and pin prick are rarely lost without discernible symptoms.

Sensory examination should be used
- as a screening test
- to assess the symptomatic patient
- to test hypotheses generated by motor examination (for example to distinguish between combined ulnar and median nerve lesions and a T1 root lesion).

Sensory examination requires considerable concentration on the part of both patient and examiner. Vibration sense and joint position sense are usually quick and easy and require little concentration so always test these first. They also allow you to assess the reliability of the patient as a sensory witness.

In all parts of sensory testing it is essential first to **teach** the patient about the test. Then perform the **test**. Finally **check** that the patient has understood and carried out the test appropriately. With all testing move from areas of sensory loss to areas of normal sensation.

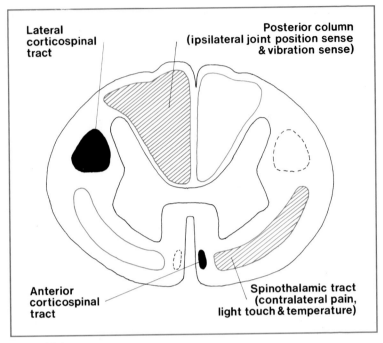

Figure 21.1
Spinal cord section showing sensory input (red) from and motor output (black) to the right side

It is important to remember that sensory signs are 'softer' than reflex or motor changes, therefore less weight is generally given to them in synthesising these findings with associated motor and reflex changes.

Arms

There are four individual nerves which are commonly affected in the arm. The relevant sensory loss is illustrated in the fingers for the median nerve, ulnar nerve, radial nerve and axillary nerve (Fig. 21.2a,b,c)

The dermatomal representation in the arms can be remembered easily if you recall that the middle finger of the hand is supplied by C7. This is illustrated in Figure 21.3.

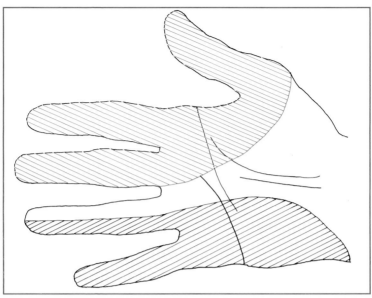

Figure 21.2a
Sensory loss in the hand: **a.** Median (red) and ulnar (black) nerves

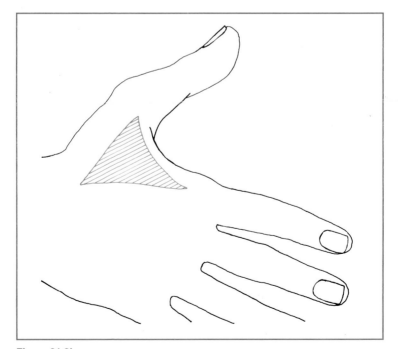

Figure 21.2b
Sensory loss in the hand: **b.** Radial nerve

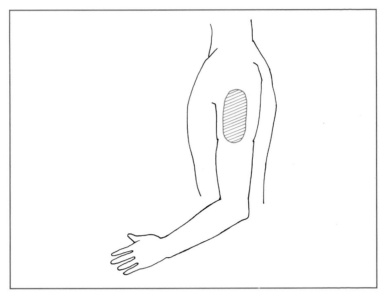

Figure 21.2c
Sensory loss in arm: **c.** Axillary nerve

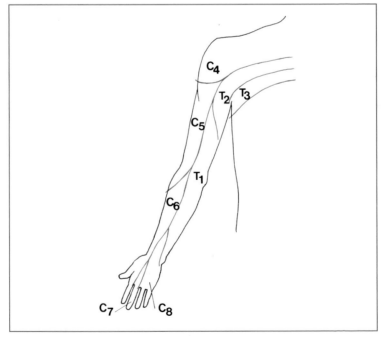

Figure 21.3
Dermatomes in the arm

Legs

Individual sensory deficit is most commonly seen in the following individual nerves:

- lateral cutaneous nerve of the thigh (Fig. 21.4a)
- common peroneal nerve (also referred to as the lateral popliteal nerve) (Fig. 21.4b)
- femoral nerve (Fig. 21.4c)
- sciatic nerve (Fig. 21.4d).

The dermatomes which are most frequently affected are L4, L5 and S1. These are illustrated in Figure 21.5.

An overview of the root innervation is given in Figure 21.6.

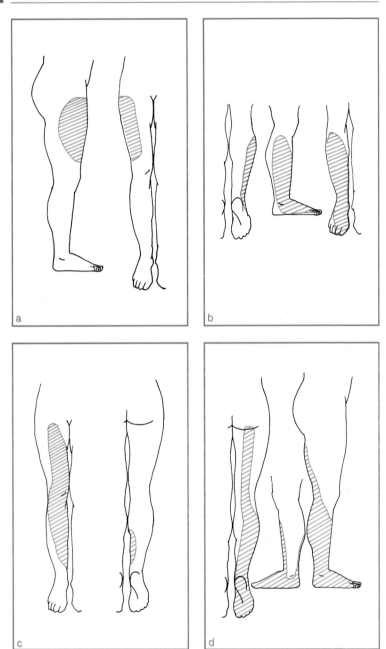

Figure 21.4
Sensory loss in the leg: **a.** Lateral cutaneous nerve of the thigh; **b.** Common peroneal nerve; **c.** Femoral nerve; **d.** Sciatic nerve

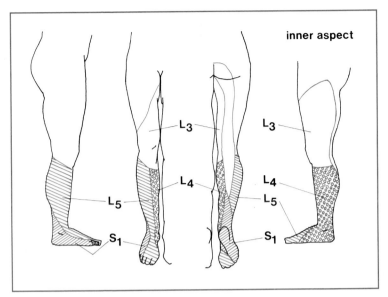

Figure 21.5
Commonly affected dermatomes in the legs

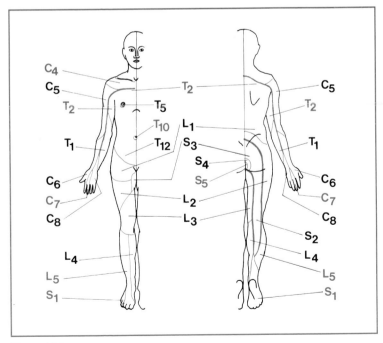

Figure 21.6
Overview of the dermatomes. Key dermatomes to remember are in red

WHAT TO DO

Vibration sense

Use a 128 Hz tuning fork. Those of higher frequency (256 or 512 Hz) are not adequate.

Demonstrate—ensure the patient understands that he is to feel a vibration, by striking the tuning fork and placing it on the sternum or chin.

Test—ask the patient to close his eyes, place the tuning fork on the bony prominence, ask if he can feel the vibration. Place initially on the toe tips then, if this is not felt, on a metatarsal phalangeal joint, medial malleolus, tibial tuberosity, anterior superior iliac spine, in the arms, on the fingertips, each interphalangeal joint, the metacarpal phalangeal joint, the wrist, the elbow and the shoulder (Fig. 21.7). If sensation is normal distally there is no point in proceeding proximally.

Check—check the patient reports feeling the vibration and not just the contact of the tuning fork. Strike the tuning fork and stop it vibrating immediately and repeat the test. If the patient reports that he feels vibration, demonstrate the test again.

N.B. Start distally and compare right with left.

Joint position sense

Demonstrate—with the patient's eyes open show him what you are going to do. Hold the distal phalanx between your two fingers (Fig. 21.8). Ensuring that your fingers are at 90° to the intended direction of movement, move the digit, illustrating which is up and which is down.

Test and check—ask the patient to close his eyes; move the toe up and down. Start with large movements in either direction; gradually reduce the angle moved until errors are made. Test distal joints first and move more proximally.

In the arm: distal proximal interphalangeal joint, middle proximal interphalangeal joint, metacarpal phalangeal joint, wrist, elbow, shoulder.

N.B. The size of movement normally detected is barely visible.

In the leg: distal interphalangeal joint, metacarpal phalangeal joint, ankle, knee and hip. N.B. Romberg's test is a test for joint position sense (see section 4).

Pin prick

Use a pin not a hypodermic needle or a broken orange stick. If a hypodermic needle is used (to be discouraged) it must be blunted before use. Dispose of the pin after use.

Try to produce a stimulus of the same intensity each time.

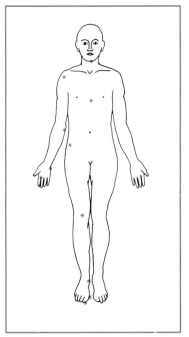

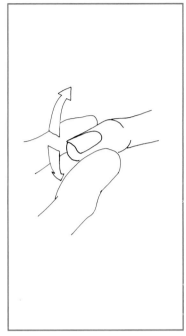

Figure 21.7
Potential sites for testing vibration
sense

Figure 21.8
How to test joint position sense

Demonstrate—show the patient what you are going to do. Explain that you want him to tell you if the pin is sharp or blunt. Touch an unaffected area with the pin and then touch an unaffected area with the opposite blunt end of the pin.

Test—ask the patient to close his eyes then apply randomly sharp and blunt stimuli and note the patient's response.

Screening test:
- start distally and move proximally. Aim to stimulate points within each dermatome and each main nerve

Assessing a lesion:
- always start from the area of altered sensation and move towards normal to find the edges.

Assessing a hypothesis:
- test within the areas of interest with great care, particularly noting any difference between the two sides.

Check—Intermittently using a blunt stimulus that needs to be recognised correctly allows you to check that the patient understands the test.

Light touch

Use a piece of cotton wool. Some people prefer to use a fingertip. Dab this on to the skin. Try to ensure a repeatable stimulus. Avoid dragging it across the skin or tickling the patient.

Demonstrate — with the patient's eyes open show him that you will be touching an area of skin. Ask him to say 'yes' every time he is touched.

Test — ask the patient to close his eyes, test the areas as for pin prick, apply the stimulus at random intervals.

Check — This is done by noting the timing of the response to the irregular stimuli. Frequently a pause of 10–20 seconds may be useful.

Special situations

Sacral sensation — this is not usually screened. However, it is essential to test sacral sensation in any patient with:

- urinary or bowel symptoms,
- bilateral leg weakness
- sensory loss in both legs
- or where a cord conus medullaris or cauda equina lesion is considered.

Common mistakes

Vibration sense and joint position sense	Inadequate explanation Hurried testing without checking
Pin prick	Drawing blood because of a non-blunted needle Varied pressure Calloused skin
Light touch	Calloused skin Varied pressure
Pin prick and cotton wool	Normal variations in sensory threshold may be interpreted as an abnormality

N.B. the ankle, the knee, the groin, the axilla are all areas of relatively heightened sensitivity

Temperature sensation

Screening

It is usually adequate to ask a patient if the tuning fork feels cold when applied to the feet and hands.

Formal testing

Fill a tube with warm water and cold water. Ideally these are controlled temperatures though normally the warm and cold tap is adequate. Dry both bottles.

Demonstrate — 'I want you to tell me if I touch you with the hot tube' (touch area of unaffected skin with the hot tube) 'or with the cold tube' (touch unaffected area of skin with the cold tube). Apply hot or cold at random to hands, feet or an affected area of interest.

Check — the random order allows assessment of concentration.

Other modalities

Two-point discrimination

This requires a two-point discriminator — a device like a blunted pair of compasses.

Demonstrate — 'I am going to touch you with either two points together' (touch an unaffected area while the patient watches with the prongs set widely apart) 'or one point' (touch with one point). 'Now close your eyes'.

Test — gradually reduce distance between prongs, touching either with one or two prongs. Note the setting at which the patient fails to distinguish one prong from two prongs.

Check — random sequence of one or two prongs allows you to assess testing.

– *Normal*: index finger < 5 mm; little finger < 7 mm; hallux < 10 mm
  N.B. varies considerably according to skin thickness
Compare right with left.

FURTHER TESTS

Sensory inattention

Ask the patient to tell you on which side you are going to touch (either with cotton wool or pinprick). Touch him on the right side and then on the left side. If he is able to recognise each independently, then touch him on both sides at the same time.

What you find
○ Recognises right, left and both normally — *normal*
○ Recognises right and left correctly but only one side, usually the right, when both stimulated — *sensory inattention*

What it means
○ Sensory inattention usually indicates a *parietal lobe lesion*, more commonly seen with lesions of the non-dominant hemisphere

WHAT YOU FIND AND WHAT IT MEANS

22

WHAT YOU FIND

Patterns of sensory loss (Flow Chart 12)

Sensory deficits can be classified into eight levels of the nervous system:

1. **Single nerve** — sensory loss within the distribution of a single nerve, most commonly median, ulnar, peroneal, lateral cutaneous nerve to the thigh. Distributions illustrated in section 21.
2. **Root or roots** — sensory deficit confined to a single root or a number of roots in close proximity: common roots in the arm C5, C6 and C7 and in the leg L4, L5 and S1. Distributions illustrated in section 21.
3. **Peripheral nerve** — distal glove and stocking deficit (Fig. 22.1).
4. **Spinal cord** — five patterns of loss can be recognised (Fig. 22.2):
   - ○ *Complete transverse lesion* — hyperaesthesia (increased appreciation of touch/pinprick) at the upper level with loss of all modalities a few segments below the lesion (Fig. 22.2a).
   - ○ *Hemisection of the cord* (Brown–Séquard syndrome) — loss of joint position sense and vibration sense on the same side as the lesion and pain and temperature on the opposite side a few levels below the lesion (Fig. 22.2b).
   - ○ *Central cord* — loss of pain and temperature, sensation at the level of the lesion, where the spinothalamic fibres cross in the cord, with other modalities preserved (dissociated sensory loss) — seen in syringomyelia (Fig. 22.2c)
   - ○ *Posterior column loss* — loss of joint position sense and vibration sense with intact pain and temperature (Fig. 22.2d).
   - ○ *Anterior spinal syndrome* — loss of pain and temperature below the level with preserved joint position sense and vibration sense (Fig. 22.2e).
5. **Brainstem**: loss of pain and temperature on the face and on the opposite side of the body — *common cause*: lateral medullary syndrome (Fig. 22.2f).
6. **Thalamic sensory loss**: hemisensory loss of all modalities (Fig. 22.2g).

Approach to sensory loss

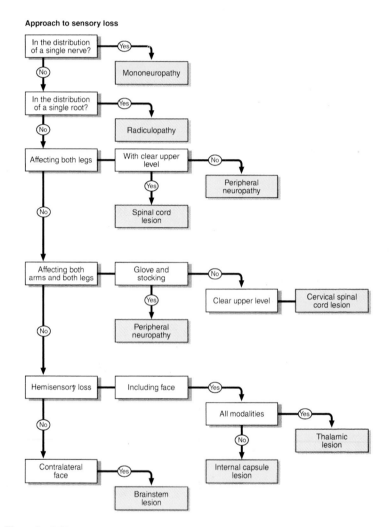

Flow chart 12
Simplified approach to sensory loss

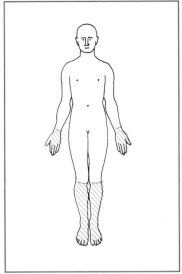

Cross section of spinal cord: lesions shaded in red. LCT = lateral corticospinal tract; ACT = anterior corticospinal tract; PC = posterior column; STT = spinothalamic tract

Sensory modalities: areas of sensory loss shaded in red. Modalities are marked: x = absent, tick = present. pp = pinprick; temp = temperature; vs = vibration sense; jps = joint position sense; lt = light touch

Figure 22.1
Glove and stocking loss

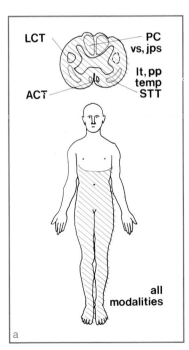

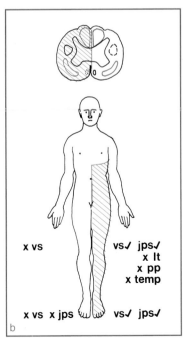

Figure 22.2a & b
Sensory loss associated with spinal cord lesions: **a.** Complete transverse lesion; **b.** Hemisection of the cord

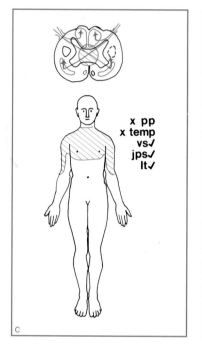

x pp
x temp
vs✓
jps✓
lt✓

c

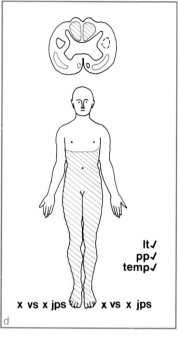

lt✓
pp✓
temp✓

x vs x jps   x vs x jps

d

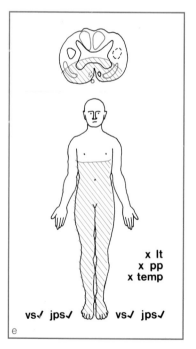

x lt
x pp
x temp

vs✓ jps✓   vs✓ jps✓

e

Figure 22.2c, d & e
c. Central cord lesion; **d.** Posterior column loss; **d.** Anterior spinal syndrome

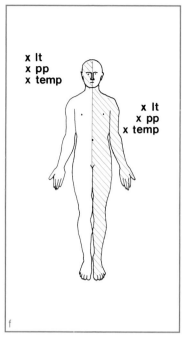
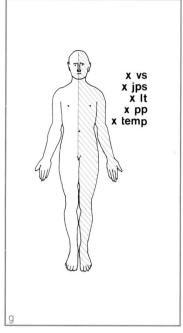

Figure 22.2f & g
f. Brainstem lesion; **g.** Thalamic sensory loss

7. **Cortical loss** — parietal lobe: the patient is able to recognise all sensations but localises them poorly — loss of two-point discrimination, astereognosis, sensory inattention.
8. **Functional loss**: this diagnosis is suggested by a non-anatomical distribution of sensory deficit frequently with inconstant findings.

WHAT IT MEANS

○ **Single nerve lesion** — *common cause*: entrapment neuropathy. More common in diabetes mellitus, rheumatoid arthritis, hypothyroidism. May be presentation of more diffuse neuropathy (see section 20)
○ **Multiple single nerve lesions**: mononeuritis multiplex — *common causes*: vasculitis, or presentation of more diffuse neuropathy
○ **Single root lesion** — *common causes*: compression by prolapsed intervertebral discs; *rare causes*: tumours (e.g. neurofibroma)
○ **Peripheral nerve** (see section 20) — *common causes*: diabetes mellitus, alcohol-related vitamin B_1 deficiency, drugs (e.g. vincristine); frequently no cause is found; *rarer causes*: Guillain–Barré syndrome, inherited neuropathies (e.g. Charcot–Marie–Tooth disease), vasculitis, other vitamin deficiencies

○ **Spinal cord**
  – **Complete transection**—*common causes*: trauma, spinal cord compression by tumour (usually bony secondaries in vertebra), cervical spondylitis, transverse myelitis, multiple sclerosis; *rare causes*: intraspinal tumours (e.g. meningiomas), spinal abscess, post-infectious (usually viral)
  – **Hemisection**—*common causes*: as for transection
  – **Central cord syndrome** (rare)—*common causes*: syringomyelia, trauma leading to haematomyelia
  – **Posterior column loss**—any cause of complete transection but also the rare subacute combined degeneration of the cord (vitamin B_{12} deficiency) and tabes dorsalis
  – **Anterior spinal syndrome** (rare)—anterior spinal artery emboli or thrombosis
○ **Brainstem pattern** (rare)—*common causes*: in young patients—demyelination, in older patients—brainstem stroke; rare causes: brainstem tumours
○ **Thalamic and cortical loss**—*common causes*: stroke (thrombosis, emboli or haemorrhage), cerebral tumour, multiple sclerosis, trauma
○ **Functional**—may indicate hysterical illness. N.B. this is a difficult diagnosis to make in the absence of appropriate psychopathology

N.B. The diverse range of aetiologies offered for each of the patterns of sensory loss reinforces the importance of the history in making sense of the clinical findings.

23

CO-ORDINATION

BACKGROUND

A co-ordinated combination of a series of motor actions is needed to produce a smooth and accurate movement. This requires integration of sensory feedback with motor output. This integration occurs mainly in the cerebellum.

In the presence of weakness tests for co-ordination must be interpreted with caution and are unlikely to be informative if there is significant weakness.

Loss of joint position sense can produce some inco-ordination (sensory ataxia). This is made substantially worse when the eyes are closed. Joint position sense should be tested before coordination.

WHAT TO DO

Test the gait (see section 4)
In all tests compare right with left. Expect the right hand to be slightly better (in a right-handed person).

Arms

Ask the patient to hold his arms outstretched and ask him to close his eyes. Tell the patient to keep his arms in this position. Then push his arm up or down suddenly.

Finger–nose test
Hold your finger out about an arm's length in front of the patient. Ask the patient to touch your finger with his index finger and then touch his nose. (Fig. 23.1) When he has done this correctly ask him to repeat this faster. The test can be made more sensitive by moving the target finger.

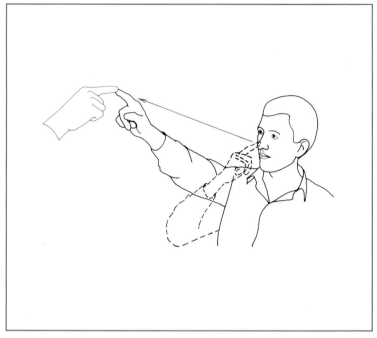

Figure 23.1
The finger-nose test

Repeated movements

Ask the patient to pat one hand on the back of the other quickly and regularly (*demonstrate*).

Ask the patient to twist his hand as if opening a door or unscrewing a light bulb (*demonstrate*).

Ask the patient to tap the back of his right hand alternately with the palm, and then the back of his left hand. Repeat with the right hand (*demonstrate*).

Legs

Heel–shin test

The patient is lying down. Ask him to lift his leg and place the point of his heel on his knee and then run it down the sharp part of his shin (Fig. 23.2) (*demonstrate*).

Common mistake

● allowing the patient to run his instep along his shin

Ask the patient to tap his feet as if listening to fast music.

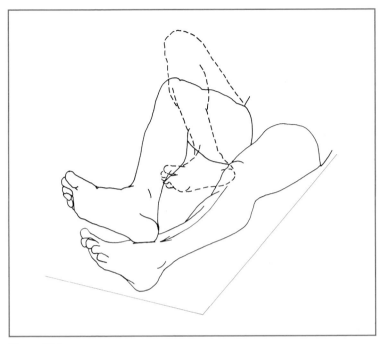

Figure 23.2
The heel-shin test

Trunk
Ask the patient to sit up from lying without using his hands
Does he fall to one side?

OTHER ABNORMALITIES OF CEREBELLAR FUNCTION

1. Speech (section 2)
2. Nystagmus (section 10)
3. Hypotonia (section 16)
4. Pendular reflexes (section 19)
5. Tremor (section 24)

WHAT YOU FIND

With outstretched arms

○ The arms oscillate several times before coming to rest — this indicates *cerebellar disease*
○ The arms return rapidly to position — *normal*

Finger–nose test

○ The patient is able to complete the task quickly and accurately — *normal*
○ The patient develops a tremor as his finger approaches its target — *intention tremor*; finger overshoots its targets — *past pointing* or *dysmetria*

Repeated movements

○ Disorganisation of the movement of the hands and the elbows taking wider excursions than expected; irregularity of the movements which are performed without rhythm. Compare the two sides — these changes indicate *cerebellar inco-ordination*. Often the abnormality is heard as a slapping sound rather than the normal tapping noise

N.B. Mild upper motor neurone weakness would impair fluency of fast repeated movements but the movements will not be of wider excursion or irregular.

When there is disorganisation of tapping the hand and then turning it over this is referred to as *dysdiadochokinesia*.

Heel–shin

○ Disorganisation of movement with the heel falling off the anterior part of the shin, knee falling from side to side

N.B. The finger–nose and heel–shin test can be used as an indication of loss of joint position sense. The original movements are accurate but when repeated with the eyes closed are substantially worse — this indicates impairment of joint position sense.

Trunk

○ Patient is unable to sit from lying without falling to one side = *truncal ataxia*. Associated with gait ataxia (section 4)

WHAT IT MEANS

○ **Unilateral inco-ordination** — ipsilateral cerebellar syndrome
○ **Bilateral inco-ordination** — bilateral cerebellar syndrome
○ **Truncal ataxia, gait ataxia, without limb inco-ordination** — midline cerebellar syndrome
○ **Unilateral cerebellar syndrome** — *common causes*: demyelination, vascular disease; *rare causes*: trauma, tumour or abscess
○ **Bilateral cerebellar syndrome** — *common causes*: drugs (anticonvulsants), alcohol, demyelination, vascular disease; *rare causes*:

hereditary cerebellar degenerations, paraneoplastic disorders, hypothyroidism
○ **Midline cerebellar syndrome**: lesion of the cerebellar vermis — *causes* as for bilateral cerebellar syndrome

24

ABNORMAL MOVEMENTS

BACKGROUND

Abnormal movements are best appreciated by seeing affected patients. Armed with the right vocabulary, most common abnormal movements can be described. However many experts will describe the same movements in different ways — so journals about movement disorders come with a video cassette to illustrate the movements!

In most patients with movement disorder the diagnosis depends on an accurate description of the clinical phenomenon.

There is frequently a considerable overlap between syndromes and several types of abnormal movement are often seen in the same patient — for example, tremor and dystonia in a parkinsonian patient on treatment.

The anatomy of the basal ganglia is complicated and the wiring diagrams illustrating the connections between the various structures get more complicated as more research is done. Neuro-anatomical correlations are of limited clinical value as most movement disorders are classified as syndromes rather than on anatomical grounds. Correlations of significance include unilateral parkinsonism due to lesions of contralateral substantia nigra and unilateral hemiballismus due to lesions of the contralateral subthalamic nucleus or its connections.

In evaluating movement disorders there are three aspects to the examination:

1. **Positive phenomena**
   - the abnormal positions maintained
   - the additional movements seen
2. **Latent phenomena**
   - the abnormal phenomena that can be revealed using various manoeuvres (e.g. rigidity on testing tone and the abnormal postures brought on by writing in writer's cramp)
3. **Negative phenomena**
   - the inability to do things, for example a slowness in initiating actions (bradykinesia)

Terms used in movement disorders (Fig. 24.1)

Akathisia — motor restlessness where the patient constantly shifts, crossing and uncrossing his legs and walking on the spot.

Athetosis — slower writhing irregular movements predominantly in the hands and wrist (used less frequently now).

Chorea — rhythmical movements of a rapid, jerky nature which frequently appear pseudo-purposeful. They may be voluntarily controlled for a short time.

Dyskinesia — a term used to describe movements associated with neuroleptic drugs; particularly used to describe movements of mouth and face (oro-facial dyskinesia).

Dystonia — co-contraction of agonist and antagonist which may lead to an intermittent or persistent maintenance of abnormal posture. Position maintained is usually at an extreme of extension or flexion.

Hemiballismus — violent and flinging movements which are irregular affecting one side. There is no clear distinction from severe chorea.

Myoclonic jerk — an extremely brief contraction of a muscle group leading to involuntary purposeless jerk of affected limb.

Tic — a stereotyped and irresistible repetitive action, normally a repeated purposeful action.

Tremor — rhythmical alternating movement

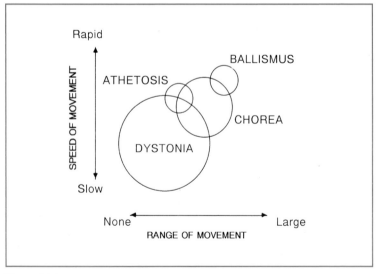

Figure 24.1
There is a considerable overlap between chorea and athetosis; chorea and hemiballismus, and chorea and dystonia

WHAT TO DO

Look at the patient's face
- are there any additional movements?
- is the face expressionless?

Look at the patient's head position

Look at the arms and the legs
- note the position
- are there any abnormal movements?

Ask the patient to:
- smile
- close his eyes
- hold hands out in front of him with his wrist cocked back (Fig. 24.2a)
- lift his elbows out sideways and point his index fingers at one another in front of his nose (Fig. 24.2b)
- perform finger–nose test (as in section 23)

If there is a tremor note the frequency, the degree of the excursion (fine, moderate, large), note body parts affected. Look for a tongue tremor (see section 13).

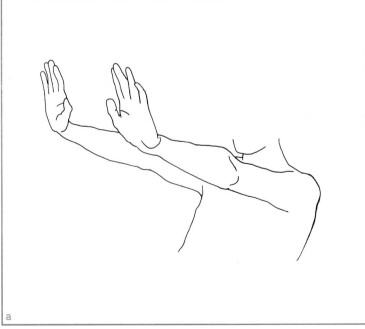

Figure 24.2a
Testing for tremor

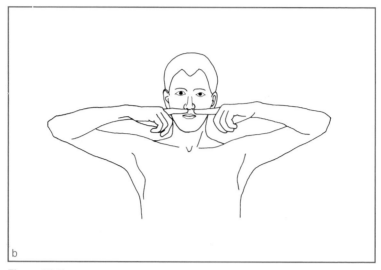

Figure 24.2b

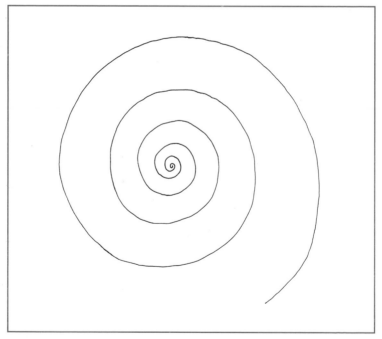

Figure 24.3
Archimedes spiral

Test eye movements (section 9)

Test tone (section 16). When testing tone in one arm it is sometimes useful to ask the patient to lift the other arm up and down.

Test fast repeating movements
Ask the patient to
- rapidly bring thumb and index finger together (*demonstrate*)
- rapidly touch the thumb with each finger in turn (*demonstrate*)
- tap his toe as if listening to fast music

Observe the speed of the movements and whether they break up.

Gait (section 4)

Writing:
Ask the patient to
- write his name and address
- draw an Archimedes spiral (Fig. 24.3)

Ask the patient to perform any manoeuvre that he reports may trigger the abnormal movement

WHAT YOU FIND

Face

Positive phenomena

Commonly
- ○ Lipsmacking and twisting of mouth — *oro-facial dyskinesia*
- ○ Flickering of muscles particularly around eye — *facial myokymia*

Rarely
- ○ Intermittent spasm of muscles around the eye — *blepharospasm*
- ○ Intermittent spasm of muscles of one side of the face — *hemifacial spasm*

Negative phenomena
- ○ Facial immobility

Head

Positive phenomena
Position
- ○ Head twisted to one side — *torticollis*
- ○ Head bent forward — *anterocollis*
- ○ Head bent backwards — *retrocollis*

Movement
- ○ Rhythmical movement of head — *titubation*: described as yes–yes (shaking forward–backwards) or no–no (side to side)

Arms and legs

Positive phenomena

Tremor

○ Present when limb (particularly hand) is at rest—*rest tremor*
○ Present when limb is maintained in a position (esp as in Fig. 24.2)—*postural tremor*
○ Present during an action (e.g. finger–nose testing)—*action tremor*
○ Present and increasing as the finger reaches its target—*intention tremor*

N.B. commonly more than one type of tremor co-exist.

Position

○ Limb maintained, often only transiently, in abnormal position with contraction of both agonists and antagonists = *dystonic posturing*. Commonly the arm is abducted at the shoulder, extended at the elbow, pronated to an extreme position with the fingers extended. The leg is usually extended at the hip and knee and inverted at the ankle with the toes flexed.

Hint: try to put yourself into these positions to realise what they look like (and why the patients find them uncomfortable).

Additional movements (as described above). Describe which part of the movements are seen to be affected.
• myoclonus
• chorea
• hemiballismus
• tic
• athetosis

Latent phenomena

On walking the following may occur or increase:
○ Rest tremor
○ Dystonic posturing
○ Chorea

Finger–nose testing may reveal
○ Action tremor
○ Intention tremor (see above)
○ Myoclonus—*action myoclonus*

and exacerbate
○ Choreic movements

Fast repeating movements
○ Slowed or break up easily—*bradykinesia*

Tone
○ Cogwheel rigidity may be found only when the other arm is lifted up and down (activated)

Writing
○ Writing becomes progressively slower, the hand may go into spasm, patient often holds pen in unusual way — writer's cramp

Archimedes spiral
○ Spiral very tight, ending up as a circle — suggests parkinsonism
○ Spiral very large with tremor — suggests cerebellar syndrome

Negative phenomena
○ Rigidity — lead-pipe or cogwheel
○ Bradykinesia — slowness in initiating movements
○ Reduced armswing on walking (see section 4)

WHAT IT MEANS
Akinetic–rigid syndromes (Parkinsonism)

○ *Key features* — rigidity, bradykinesia and tremor
Features include reduced facial expression (mask like), rest tremor, stooped posture with reduced armswing and increased tremor on walking. Gait may be festinant (section 4). Bradykinesia on fast repeating movements and walking. Extrapyramidal dysarthria (section 2). May be limitation of convergence. Glabellar tap positive (not useful).
○ *Common causes* — Parkinson's disease, major tranquilliser (e.g. chlorpromazine, haloperidol)
○ *Rare causes* — Steele–Richardson syndrome (akinetic–rigid syndrome associated with progressive supranuclear palsy), multiple systems atrophy (akinetic rigid syndrome associated with autonomic failure), Wilson's disease

Tremors

○ **Rest tremor** — feature of akinetic rigid syndrome (see above)
○ **Postural and action tremor** — *common causes*: benign essential tremor (also called familial tremor if there is a family history), exaggerated physiological tremor (may be caused by hyper-thyroidism, beta-agonists) — *rarer causes*: liver failure, renal failure, alcohol withdrawal
○ **Intention tremor** — indicates cerebellar disease (see section 23)

Chorea

Common causes
○ Drug therapy of Parkinson's disease (excess treatment)

Rare causes
- ○ Wilson's disease (look for associated liver disease and Keyser Fleisher rings on cornea)
- ○ Huntington's disease (trace family history)
- ○ Post-pill or pregnancy chorea
- ○ Sydenham's chorea
- ○ Stroke

Hemiballismus

- ○ Lesion of the contralateral subthalamic nucleus or its connections — *common cause*: stroke

Dystonia

Affects only one part of the body — **focal dystonia**
- ○ Isolated torticollis
- ○ Isolated writer's cramp

Affecting two or more adjacent parts of the body — **segmental dystonia**. For example
- ○ Torticollis and dystonic posturing in the same arm

Affects parts of the body that are not adjacent
- ○ **Generalised dystonia**: often associated with chorea

Common causes
- ○ **Focal and segmental dystonia** — idiopathic, major tranquillisers, treated Parkinson's disease on excessive therapy
- ○ **Generalised dystonia** — as for chorea above — *rare causes*: dystonia musculorum deformans

Tic

Usually an isolated finding, may be associated with coprolalia (muttering of obscenities); referred to then as Gilles de la Tourette syndrome.

Myoclonic jerk

May be seen as part of other movement disorders where chorea or dystonia is predominant.

Associated with a number of metabolic encephalopathies, myoclonic epilepsies — seen in rare neurological diseases such as Creutzfeldt–Jakob disease and postanoxic encephalitis.

Others

- **Oro-facial dyskinesia**—usually a late reaction to major tranquilliser. May also occur as part of the syndromes listed under chorea
- **Akathisia**—late reaction to major tranquilliser
- **Blepharospasm**—idiopathic
- **Hemifacial spasm**—compression of facial nerve by ectopic vessels
- **Facial myokymia**—usually benign, possibly exacerbated by tiredness, caffeine; *rarely*: indicative of brainstem lesion

25

SPECIAL SIGNS

In this section are a number of signs which are used on particular occasions:
1. Primitive reflexes
2. Superficial reflexes
3. Tests for meningeal irritation
4. Miscellaneous tests

1. PRIMITIVE REFLEXES

Snout reflex

What you do
Ask the patient to close his eyes, tap his mouth gently with a patella hammer.

What you find
○ No reaction — *normal*
○ Puckering of lips — *positive snout reflex*

Palmo-mental reflex

What you do
Scratch the palm of the patient's hand briskly across the centre of the palm and look at the chin.

What you find
○ No reaction — *normal*
○ Contraction of a muscle on the same side of the chin — *positive palmo-mental reflex*

Grasp reflex

What you do
Place your fingers on the patient's palm and pull your hand away, asking the patient to let go of your hand.

What you find
○ The patient is able to let go — *normal*
○ Patient involuntarily grabs your hand — *positive grasp reflex*

What it means

All these primitive reflexes may be found in normals. They occur more frequently in patients with frontal pathology and diffuse encephalopathy. If unilateral they strongly suggest contralateral frontal lobe pathology.

2. SUPERFICIAL REFLEXES

Cremasteric reflex

This reflex can be performed in men. The inner aspect of the upper thigh is stroked downward. The movement of the testicle in the scrotum is watched. Cremasteric contraction elevates the testicle that side.
Afferent: femoral nerve L1, L2
Efferent: L1, L2

What you find
Absent — may occur with non-neurological local pathology or previous local surgery
— lesion in reflex arc
— pyramidal lesion above L1

Anal reflex

What you do
Lie the patient on his side with the knees flexed. Lightly stroke the anal margin with an orange stick.

What you find
○ Visible contraction of the external anal sphincter

What it means
This tests the integrity of the reflex arc with segmental elevation of S4 and S5 for sensory and motor components.

3. TESTS FOR MENINGEAL IRRITATION

Neck stiffness

What to do

N.B. Not to be performed if there could be cervical instability — e.g. following trauma or in patients with rheumatoid arthritis.

The patient should be lying flat.

Place your hands behind the patient's head

- gently rotate the head — moving the head as if the patient was indicating no. Feel the stiffness
- gently lift the head off the bed — feel the tone in the neck
- watch the legs for hip and knee flexion

What you find and what it means

○ Neck moves easily in both planes, with the chin easily reaching the chest on neck flexion — *normal*
○ Neck rigid on movement — **neck stiffness**
  - Indicates: meningeal irritation — *common causes*: viral and bacterial meningitis, subarachnoid haemorrhage — rarer causes: carcinomatous, granulomatous, fungal meningitis
  - May also occur in: severe cervical spondylosis, parkinsonism, with tonsillar herniation
  N.B. proceed to test for Kernig's sign
○ Hip and knee flexion in response to neck flexion = Brudzinski's sign (Fig. 25.1). This indicates meningeal irritation

Hint: Cervical lymphadenopathy and severe pharyngitis may simulate neck stiffness — but stiffness is usually only on flexion and appropriate physical signs of these pathologies are easily found.

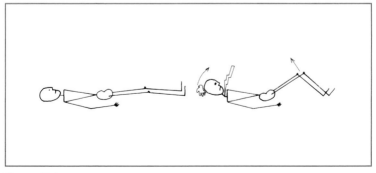

Figure 25.1
Brudzinski's sign

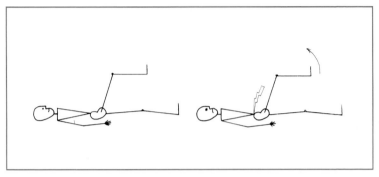

Figure 25.2
Kernig's sign

Testing for Kernig's sign

What to do
The patient is lying flat on the bed.
- flex the leg at the hip with the knee flexed
- then try to extend the knee
- repeat on the other side (Fig. 25.2).

What you find
- ○ Knee straightens without difficulty — *normal*
- ○ Resistance to knee straightening — *Kernig's sign*: indicates meningeal irritation or, if unilateral, may occur with radiculopathy (cf straight leg raising).

N.B. Kernig's sign is absent with other causes of neck stiffness.

4. MISCELLANEOUS TESTS AND SIGNS

Tinel's test
Percussion of a nerve at putative site of compression (usually using a tendon hammer). It is positive when paraesthesiae are produced in the distribution of the nerve concerned. Commonly performed to test for median nerve compression at the wrist.

Lhermitte's phenomenon

Forward flexion of the neck produces an electric shock feeling, usually running down the back. The patient may complain of this spontaneously or you can test for it by flexing the neck. Occasionally patients have the same feeling on extension (reverse Lhermitte's).

Indicates *cervical pathology* — usually demyelination. Occasionally occurs with cervical spondylitic myelopathy or cervical tumours.

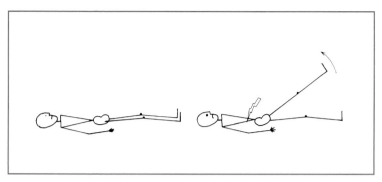

Figure 25.3
Straight leg raising

Straight leg raising (Fig. 25.3)

Test for radicular entrapment
With the patient lying flat on the bed, **lift the leg, holding the heel**.
Note angle attained and any difference between the two sides
❍ *Normal* > 90°, less in older patients
❍ Limitation with pain in back = *nerve root entrapment*

26

THE AUTONOMIC NERVOUS SYSTEM

BACKGROUND

The autonomic nervous system is made up of the sympathetic and parasympathetic nervous system.

Sympathetic system: ALARM system

Stimulation produces: tachycardia, dilatation of the bronchi, release of adrenaline and noradrenaline (maintains BP), decrease in bowel motility, inhibition of micturition (stimulates internal urethral sphincter, relaxes detrusor muscle), increase in sweating and dilation of the pupils. (Remember what happens when you go into an exam.)

Parasympathetic system: HOLIDAY system

Stimulation produces: bradycardia, constriction of the bronchi, increase in salivation and lacrimation, increase in bowel motility, erections, initiation of micturition (relaxes the internal urethral sphincter, contraction of detrusor) and constriction of the pupils.

Outflow

- *sympathetic system* — T1–L2
- *parasympathetic system* — cranial nerves III, VII, IX and X, and S2–4

Bedside testing of the autonomic nervous system is limited.

Patterns of bladder and bowel disturbance are outlined separately (see box)

WHAT TO DO

Examine the pupils (see section 7)

Take the resting pulse
- check pulse when asking patients to take 10 breaths per minute
- estimate difference between maximum and minimum rate (ideally done using ECG monitoring).

Check pulse response to standing (for 15 beats)

Ask the patient to take a deep breath and exhale against a closed glottis—a Valsalva manoeuvre (you will probably have to demonstrate this)—and then ask the patient to breath normally. Note the effect the Valsalva and release has on the pulse

Take the lying and standing blood pressure

Look at the colour of the skin and note any sweating

Feel the skin temperature

WHAT YOU FIND
Pupils

- Horner's syndrome (ptosis, meiosis, enophthalmos, anhydrosis)—*sympathetic defect*
- Sluggish reactions to light and accommodation—*autonomic neuropathy*

Pulse and BP tests

. Test	Normal	Abnormalities found
Resting pulse	60–100	Tachycardia—PARAS abnormal
Heart rate response to respiration 10/min	Max-min >15/min	Loss of variation—PARAS abnormal
Heart rate response to standing (1st 15 beats)	>11/min increase	Loss of response—PARAS abnormal
BP response to standing	Fall <30/15	Increased drop'—SYMP abnormal
Heart rate response to Valsalva	HR up during	HR stable during—SYMP abnormal
	HR down after	HR stable after—PARAS abnormal

Abbreviations SYMP = sympathetic system, PARAS = parasympathetic, HR = heart rate

Skin

- Red and hot with impaired sweating—*sympathetic lesion*

WHAT IT MEANS

○ **Horner's syndrome** — see section 7.
○ **Autonomic neuropathy** — *common cause*: diabetes mellitus; *rare causes*: Guillain–Barré syndrome, amyloidosis, multisystem atrophy (also called Shy–Drager syndrome — see section 24), orthostatic hypotension, congenital autonomic failure (Riley–Day syndrome)
○ **Localised sympathetic lesions** — surgical sympathectomy

Common mistakes

• drugs can interfere with autonomic function tests: e.g. betablockers and agents with anticholinergic action block parts of the autonomic nervous system
• general medical conditions such as pneumonia or anaemia will affect the cardiovascular response and interfere with autonomic testing

---

Bladder and bowel function

Patterns of abnormality

Frontal bladder
○ Urinary urgency, precipitant and uncontrolled voiding of large volumes without residual urine. Periods of urinary control. Normal anal tone. Frontal release signs (section 25)
Occurs in dementia, normal pressure hydrocephalus, frontal tumours

Spinal bladder
○ Initially urinary retention ± overflow incontinence. Later bladder contracts and voids small volumes of urine automatically and precipitantly. Constipation. Normal anal tone. May develop reflex penile erections — called priapism (after the Greek god Priapus)
○ *Occurs in* spinal cord lesions — *common causes*: trauma, multiple sclerosis, spinal tumour

Peripheral neurogenic bladder
○ Painless distention of flaccid bladder with overflow incontinence and large residual volumes. Faecal incontinence. Reduced anal tone. There may be saddle anaesthesia. Impotence
○ *Occurs in* cauda equina lesions — *common causes*: central lumbar disc protrusion; *rarer causes*: spina bifida, ependymomas, cordomas, metastases — or peripheral nerve lesions — *common causes*: diabetes mellitus; *rarer causes*: pelvic surgery, malignancy

27

THE UNCONSCIOUS PATIENT

BACKGROUND

Level of consciousness: the assessment of the unconscious and confused patient

The reticular activating system in the brainstem maintains normal consciousness. Processes that disturb its function will lead to altered consciousness.

This can happen as a result of:
1. **Diffuse encephalopathy** — generalised disturbance of brain function affecting the whole brain, including the reticular activating system
2. **Supratentorial lesions** — either massive lesions or those associated with distortion of the brainstem — 'coning' (see below)
3. **Infratentorial lesions** — producing direct damage to the brainstem.

Assessment of patients with altered consciousness will be divided into:
a. *resuscitation* (including some examination to allow you to know how to resuscitate)
b. *examination*.

Examination of unconscious patient must
- describe in a repeatable way the level of consciousness, so it can be compared with other observers' results
- distinguish the three syndromes 1–3 above
- attempt to define a cause — frequently requires further investigations.

The terms used to describe levels of unconsciousness — drowsiness, confusion, stuporous, comatose — are in everyday language and are used in different senses by different observers. It is therefore better to describe the level of consciousness individually in the terms described below.

Changes in level of consciousness and associated physical signs are very important and need to be monitored. Always record findings.

The Glasgow Coma scale is a quick, simple reliable method for monitoring level of consciousness. It includes three measures: eye opening, best motor response and best verbal response.

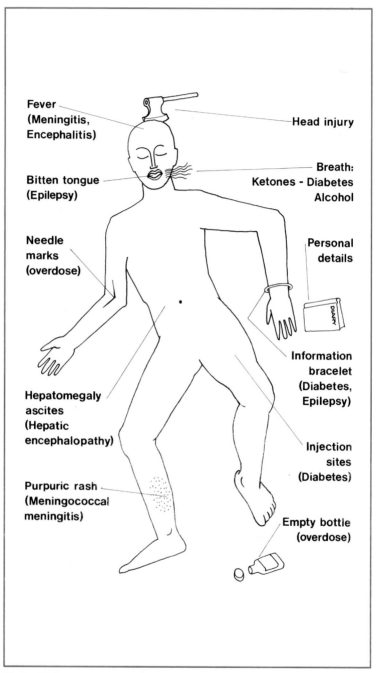

Figure 27.1
Clues to diagnosis in the unconscious patient

History can be obtained in patients with altered consciousness — either from friends, relatives, bystanders or nursing or ambulance staff. The clothing (incontinent?), jewellery (alert bracelets/necklaces), wallet and belongings are silent witnesses that may help (Fig. 27.1).

Herniation or coning

Coning is what occurs when part of the brain is forced through a rigid hole — either:

1. the uncus and the temporal lobe through the cerebellar tentorium (which separates the cerebrum from the cerebellum) = *uncal herniation*, or
2. the cerebrum is pushed centrally through the tentorium = *central herniation*.

There is a characteristic progression of signs in both types of herniation.

N.B. The signs of herniation are superimposed on top of signs due to the supratentorial mass causing the coning and are progressive.

1. Uncal herniation

What happens: A unilateral mass forces the ipsilateral temporal lobe through the tentorium compressing the ipsilateral third nerve and later the contralateral upper brainstem, and eventually the whole brainstem. Once CSF flow is interrupted the process is accelerated by an increase in intracranial pressure.

Physical signs:

Early – Ipsilateral dilated pupil and signs of supra-tentorial mass lesion

Later – Ipsilateral hemiplegia
    – Progressive ptosis and third nerve palsy
    – Cheyne–Stokes respiration

Later – Tetraparesis
    – Bilateral fixed dilated pupils
    – Erratic respiration
    – Death

Progression is usually rapid

(Continued overleaf)

2. Central herniation

What happens: A supratentorial lesion forces the diencephalon (the thalamus and related structures that lie between the upper brainstem and cerebral hemispheres) centrally through the tentorium. This compresses first the upper midbrain, later the pons and medulla.

Physical signs:

Early – Erratic respirations
– Small reactive pupils
– Increased limb tone
– Bilateral extensor plantars

Later – Cheyne–Stokes respiration
– Decorticate rigidity

Later – Fixed dilated pupils
– Decerebrate posturing

Progression usually slower

WHAT TO DO

Resuscitation

Use the Neurological ABC

N — *Neck*	Always remember there may be a neck injury. If this is possible do not manipulate the neck
A — *Airway*	Ensure there is an adequate airway, best protected by putting the patient in the recovery position
B — *Breathing*	Ensure the patient is breathing sufficiently to provide adequate oxygenation (including blood gases if necessary). Give oxygen, artificial respiration if needed
C — *Circulation*	Check there is adequate circulation, check pulse and blood pressure
D — *Diabetes*	Check the blood sugar—Destrostix, BM sticks—if not available give 50 ml 50% dextrose if the altered consciousness could be due to hypoglycaemia
— *Drugs*	Consider opiate overdose—give naloxone if indicated
E — *Epilepsy*	Observe for seizures or stigmata, bitten tongue: Control seizures

F — *Fever*   Check for fever, stiff neck, purpuric rash of meningococcal meningitis

G — *Glasgow coma scale*   Assess score out of 15 (see box)

H — *Herniation*   Is there evidence of coning? See box — rapid neurosurgical assessment

I   — *Investigate*

N.B. Pulse, BP, Respiration rate and pattern, check temperature. Monitor Glasgow coma scale.

Glasgow coma scale

	Score
Eyes open	
Never	1
To pain	2
To verbal stimuli	3
Spontaneously	4
Best verbal response	
No response	1
Incomprehensible sounds	2
Inappropriate words	3
Disorientated and converses	4
Orientated and converses	5
Best motor response	
No response	1
Extension (decerebrate rigidity) (Fig. 27.2b)	2
Abnormal flexion (decorticate rigidity) (Fig. 27.2a)	3
Flexion — withdrawal to pain	4
Localises pain	5
Obeys commands	6
Total	**15**

EXAMINATION

This is aimed at
- finding or excluding focal neurological abnormalities
- looking for evidence of meningism
- determining the level of consciousness and neurological function

Position and movement

What to do

Look at the patient — often best done from the end of the bed
- is the patient lying still *or moving*?
  If there is movement:
- are all four limbs moved equally?
- is the patient lying symmetrically?
- are there any abnormal movements?

What you find

○ Arms flexed at elbow and wrist and legs extended at knee and ankle — *decorticate posturing* (Fig. 27.2a)

○ Arms extended at elbow, pronated and flexed at wrist and legs extended at knee and ankle — *decerebrate posturing* (Fig. 27.2b)

○ Head falls to one side, with flexion of the arm — indicates *hemiparesis*

○ There are brief spasms, lasting less than a second, of arms or legs — *myoclonus*

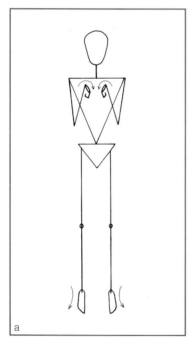
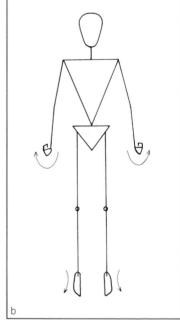

Figure 27.2a & b
Abnormal posturing

Best verbal responses

What to do

Try and rouse the patient.
• is the patient rousable?

Ask a simple question: 'What is your name?'
If you get a reply:

See if he is oriented
• in **time**: What day is it? What is the date? What is the month, year? What is the season? What is the time of day?
• in **place**: What is the name of the place we are in? What is the name of the ward/hospital? What is the name of the town/city?
• in **person**: What is your name? What job does that person do (pointing to a nurse)? What job do I do?
Make a note of the errors made

If you get no reply: try other questions: 'What happened to you?', 'Where do you live?' Note responses

What you find

Note best level of response:
• oriented
• confused conversation — using long or short sentences
• inappropriate words
• incomprehensible sounds
• none

Common mistakes: aphasia, either receptive or expressive, may be missed — giving a false level of consciousness and missing a focal dominant hemisphere sign (see section 2).

Head and neck

What to do and what you find

• inspect the head for evidence of trauma
• percuss the skull (as for chest percussion): a fracture may be associated with a 'cracked pot sound'
• look at ears and nose for evidence of CSF or bleeding. Examine the eardrums for evidence of otitis media
• test the neck for stiffness (section 25)

Do not test, if there is evidence of trauma, until cervical injury is excluded.

Eyelids

What to do and what you find
Look at the eyelids
- do they open and close spontaneously?
- tell the patient to open/close his eyes
- assess response to pain—do eyes close?
- is there any eyelid movement?

Is the eyelid movement symmetrical?
- is there a ptosis?
- is there a facial weakness?

Pupils

What to do
Look at the pupils
- note size in mm
- test direct and consensual light reflexes (see section 7)

What you find

Pupils equal	pinpoint		*opiates* or *pontine lesion*
	small	reactive	*metabolic encephalopathy*
	mid-sized	fixed	*midbrain lesion*
		reactive	*metabolic lesion*
Pupils unequal	dilated	unreactive	*IIIrd palsy*
	small	reactive	*Horner's syndrome*

Fundi

Examine the fundi (section 8)
Look especially for optic nerve head swelling (rare), or subhyaloid haemorrhages

Common mistake
- *absence* of papilloedema does not exclude raised intracranial pressure

Eye movements

What to do
Watch the eye movements
- do they look at you?
- do they follow a moving object, such as a torch?

- do they move together (conjugately) or independently (disconjugately)?
- do they move at all?
- what is their position?

Test doll's eye manoeuvre (see below)

What you find
○ skew deviation: *brainstem lesion*
  If the patient can follow objects
○ test eye movements as in section 9
○ evidence of third, fourth or sixth nerve palsies, lateral gaze palsy
  (see section 9 and consider uncal herniation)

Oculocephalic testing of eye movements (doll's eye manoeuvre):

What to do

(N.B. Not to be done unless cervical injury is excluded)

Turn the head to the right
Watch the eyes
- do they both turn to the left?
- do they keep looking ahead
- does one move and not the other?

Test the other side and neck extension and flexion

What you find:
○ Eyes move in the opposite direction to head movement — as if trying to look straight: *normal*
○ Yes move to one side but not the other: *lateral gaze palsy* — brainstem lesion
○ Limitation of abduction of one eye: *VI nerve palsy*
○ Limitation of movements other than abduction in one eye with dilated pupil: *III nerve palsy*
○ Eyes fail to move in any direction — *bilateral brainstem lesions*

Caloric test: see section 12

Corneal reflex: see section 11

Gag reflex: see section 13

Motor system

What to do

Assess the tone in all four limbs (section 16)
- is it symmetrical?

Assess the movement in each limb
Look at the spontaneous movements of the limbs
- are they symmetrical?

Ask the patient to move the limb
If he co-operates: test power more formally
If no response:

Press the knuckle of your thumb into the sternum
- is there a purposeful movement to the site of pain?
- do arms flex with this pain?
- do arms and legs extend with pain?
- is there asymmetry in these responses?
If no response to this stimulus:
Apply pressure to inner end of eyebrow. Note response
Squeeze the nail bed of a digit in each limb: does limb withdraw?

Tendon reflexes

See section 19.

Are they symmetrical?
Plantar response: extensor or flexor

What you find

○ Best motor response is found:
- – Obeys commands
- – Localises
- – Withdraws
- – Abnormal flexion
- – Extension response
- – None

○ Record abnormal responses for each limb
○ Asymmetry in tone, reflexes or response to pain: indicates *hemiparesis*

WHAT YOU FIND AND WHAT IT MEANS

Patients with coma can be classified into one of the following groups:

1. Patients without focal signs
   a. Without signs of meningism
   b. With meningism
2. Patients with focal signs indicative of either central herniation or uncal herniation (supratentorial lesions)

3. Patients with brainstem signs not indicative of coning (infratentorial lesions)

In most patients accurate diagnosis depends on appropriate further investigations — these investigations are given in brackets for the common causes of coma.

COMMON CAUSES OF COMA

The most common are marked with an asterisk

1. Diffuse and multifocal processes

a. Without meningism

Metabolic
- *Hypoglycaemia (blood glucose)
- *Hyperglycaemia (blood glucose)
- *Hypoxia (blood gases)
- *Acidosis (blood gases)
- Thiamine deficiency 'Wernicke's encephalopathy'
- Hepatic failure
- Renal failure
- Hypercapnia (excess CO_2)
- Hypoadrenalism

Toxin-induced
- **Drugs — benzodiazepines, barbiturates, opiates, tricyclics (toxicology screen)
- *Alcohol (toxicology)

Infectious
- *Encephalitis — Herpes simplex and other viruses (CSF examination, EEG)

Vascular
- Hypertensive encephalopathy

Trauma
- *Concussion (CT brain)

Epilepsy
- *Post-ictal

Temperature regulation
- Hypothermia (rectal temperature)

b. With meningism

Vascular
- *Subarachnoid haemorrhage (CT brain, CSF examination)
  N.B. may have focal signs — brainstem or hemisphere

Infections
○ Meningitis—bacterial and viral (blood cultures, CT scan, CSF examination and culture)

2. Supratentorial lesions (CT brain)

○ Haemorrhage
  - Extradural
  - *Subdural
  - *Intracerebral
○ Infarction
  - Embolic
  - Thrombotic
○ Tumours
  - Primary
  - Secondary
  - Abscess

3. Subtentorial lesions (CT brain)

○ Haemorrhage
  - Cerebellar
  - Pontine
○ Infarction
  - Brainstem
○ Tumours
  - Cerebellum
○ Abscess
  - Cerebellum

28

SUMMARY OF SCREENING NEUROLOGICAL EXAMINATION

If the history reveals no suggestion of focal neurological deficit, no speech disturbance and no disturbance of higher function, then you can use a screening neurological examination.

Screening neurological examination

- ○ **Gait**
- ○ **Pupils** — direct and consensual reactions
- ○ **Test fields** to hand movements
- ○ **Fundoscopy**
- ○ **Eye movements** to pursuit on upgaze and lateral gaze
- ○ **Facial sensation** to light touch with finger tip in all three divisions of trigeminal
- ○ **Facial movement** — 'screw up your eyes — show me your teeth'
- ○ **Mouth** — 'open your mouth' (look at tongue) 'and say "ahh" (observe palate). 'Please put out your tongue.'
- ○ **Test neck flexion**
- ○ **Arms**
  - look for wasting
  - test tone at wrist and elbow
  - observe outstretched arms with eyes closed (pronator test)
  - test power (shoulder abduction, elbow flexion and extension, finger extension and abduction and abductor pollicis brevis)
  - reflexes (biceps, triceps and supinator)
- ○ **Legs**
  - look for wasting
  - test tone at hip
  - test power (hip flexion and extension, knee flexion and extension, foot dorsiflexion and plantar flexion)
  - reflexes (knee, ankle and plantar response)
- ○ **Sensation**
  - test joint position sense in toes and fingers
  - test vibration sense on toes and fingers
  - test light touch and pinprick distally in hand and feet.
- ○ **Coordination** — test finger–nose and heel–shin

BIBLIOGRAPHY FOR FURTHER READING AND REFERENCE

Further information about the neurological conditions mentioned in this book can be obtained in the standard textbooks listed below. More detailed information relating to the examination of the peripheral nervous system and general examination can be obtained from the reference sources and books on general examination given below.

Small neurology textbooks

Perkin GD 1986 Basic neurology. Ellis Horwood, Chichester
Patten J 1977 Neurological differential diagnosis. Springer-Verlag, New York
Lindsay KW, Bone I, Callander R 1986 Neurology and neurosurgery illustrated. Churchill Livingstone, Edinburgh

Large neurology textbooks

Adams RD, Victor M 1989 Principles of neurology, 4th edn. McGraw-Hill, New York
Walton J 1985 Brain's diseases of the nervous system, 9th edn. Oxford University Press, Oxford

Very large neurology textbooks

Swash M, Oxbury J (eds) 1991 Clinical neurology. Churchill Livingstone, Edinburgh
Bradley WG, Daroff RB, Fenichel GM, Marsden CD (eds) 1991 Neurology in clinical practice. Butterworth-Heinemann, Boston

Reference sources

1986 Aids to the examination of the peripheral nervous system. Eastbourne, Baillière Tindall
Devinsky O, Feldmann E 1988 Examination of the cranial and peripheral nerves. Churchill Livingstone, Edinburgh

General examination

Macleod J 1990 Clinical examination, 8th edn. Churchill Livingstone, Edinburgh

INDEX